Praise for *There I Am*

"It's moving, heartfelt, and truly inspiring."
—Cheryl Strayed, author of *Wild* and *Tiny Beautiful Things*

"Ruthie is a gifted storyteller with the unique ability to make you feel her emotions as if they're your own. Her book is somehow both bold and tender and utterly, truthfully, authentically her. She doesn't hide from heartbreak or fail to experience the fullness of all the beauty life can hold."
—Rachel Hollis, #1 *New York Times* bestselling author of
Girl, Wash Your Face and *Girl, Stop Apologizing*

"Ruthie Lindsey's voice speaks directly to the heart. *There I Am* is a testament to the things that break us, heal us, and make us who we are."
—Glennon Doyle, author of the #1 *New York Times* bestseller
Love Warrior and founder of Together Rising

"Ruthie has polished and shined and chiseled her great big life into this precious jewel for us. . . . Reading her phenomenal memoir is like going on a walk with a best friend and listening to a life-changing speech at the same time: it's equal parts familiar and profound, warm and insightful, comforting and challenging, relatable and unlike anything you've read before."
—Mari Andrew, *New York Times* bestselling author of
Am I There Yet?

"This book is an incredible gift. One of the most moving life stories I've ever read. Or heard of. It has reframed how I see pain, death, and the whole experience of life. I immediately put it up there with the great memoirs *The Glass Castle*, *Wild*, and *Educated*."

—Jedidiah Jenkins, *New York Times* bestselling author of *To Shake the Sleeping Self*

"Consistently readable and inspirational, Lindsey keeps readers in suspense about whether she will be able to fully enjoy her life. At the end, the author addresses readers directly and asks them to focus on healing what is broken in their own lives. Illness memoirs from noncelebrities often get lost in the stacks. This one deserves greater attention."

—*Kirkus Reviews*

"Compelling . . . with vibrant prose and candor . . . A harrowing and inspiring tale."

—*Booklist*

"Riveting . . . Lindsey's prose flows fluidly, and readers will be arrested by her descriptions of dealing with grief and the nature of love. . . . This inspiring story of a young woman's personal battle serves as a reminder of human resilience and hope."

—*Publishers Weekly*

"[An] unvarnished look at possibility from an earnest and openhearted writer."

—*Garden & Gun*

"Lindsey has a lesson for all of us about how easy it is to sleepwalk through the best parts of life. . . . *There I Am* is more than a story of recovery. It is a journey towards truth, the kind that will not collapse under suffering or discourage the pursuit of joy."

—Chapter16.org

There I Am

THE JOURNEY FROM HOPELESSNESS TO HEALING

RUTHIE LINDSEY

G

GALLERY BOOKS

NEW YORK LONDON TORONTO SYDNEY NEW DELHI

G

Gallery Books
An Imprint of Simon & Schuster, Inc.
1230 Avenue of the Americas
New York, NY 10020

First Gallery Books trade paperback edition April 2021

GALLERY BOOKS and colophon are registered
trademarks of Simon & Schuster, Inc.

For information about special discounts for bulk purchases,
please contact Simon & Schuster Special Sales at 1-866-506-1949
or business@simonandschuster.com.

The Simon & Schuster Speakers Bureau can bring authors
to your live event. For more information or to book an event, contact
the Simon & Schuster Speakers Bureau at 1-866-248-3049
or visit our website at www.simonspeakers.com.

Interior design by Michelle Marchese

Manufactured in the United States of America

1 3 5 7 9 10 8 6 4 2

Library of Congress Cataloging-in-Publication Data is available.

ISBN 978-1-9821-0791-8
ISBN 978-1-9821-0792-5 (pbk)
ISBN 978-1-9821-0793-2 (ebook)

For Laura Treppendahl. My precious Laura, you showed me what real abundant love looks like and any time a person feels that love from me, they are seeing a piece of you. Thank you for teaching me how to heal and for always being with me.

For Daddy, my sweet papa, you gave me my eyes. You showed me the richness of green grass and dirt and simple acts of kindness. You taught me to seek out those in need of love and protection and you filled me up with more joy than I could contain. Because of you, I know a world where love grows wild. You're the hero in this story and I carry you with me everywhere I go.

Preface

Hello, my sweet brothers and sisters.

You should know, before you read anything else, that my memory is not perfect. Once, growing up, when my brother Tim was leaving the room, he and my daddy decided to figure out exactly how much they loved each other.

"I love you," Tim said, leaving.

"I love you more," my daddy said back to him.

"No, I love *you* more." (This might be the most defiant thing Tim has ever said, by the way.)

They went back and forth for a while, and then finally my daddy asked, "How much?"

And Tim, who was born a wise and ancient soul, came up with the most expansive measurement he could for the most immeasurable love he'd known: "More than God can count."

Somewhere along the way, after hearing this sweet story a hundred times and letting it settle into my heart, I absorbed it into my own history. I decided that the entire exchange occurred between my daddy and me, not Tim.

I started saying it all the time.

I retold the story as though it were my own.

I was so sure about it that after my daddy died, *I* had *More than God Can Count* tattooed on my forearm as a memorial to him.

Years later, after I'd shared this precious phrase with the world and my tattoo artist, Tim gently informed me that it was *he* who had originally said it, not me.

This book is my best remembrance of what happened, but my memories may not be perfect. To somebody else, this story might look a little different.

Speaking of somebody elses, the people and places in these pages have shaped me. They've showed up for me and they've failed me. They've covered me in love and filled me with doubt, delivered to me my greatest joys and most immense grief. I love all of them. I'm indebted to all of them. Because this is a book about healing, because the truth I set out to tell doesn't care if somebody is called Mallory or Kate, I've chosen to give some of the beloved characters new names, and some of the details in my story have been changed. Don't worry, none of the new names are too silly.

When you've read the final page of this book and turned off your light, or gotten off at your stop, or finished the last of your coffee, I want you to forget about me, my name, my face, my journey, and look inward toward yourself. This is a story about healing, not just mine, but ours. Healing is alive in all of us, it's for all of us. I know this, feel it, in every perfect breath I take. I hope that when you're through, you'll know too.

Thank you for making space in your full, busy hearts for this story. Your time is so valued and I'm beyond grateful that you're choosing to spend some of it with me. You are loved, you are love, and I believe that healing is for you.

Prologue

I don't know why everyone's crying.

They stand over me and look down on me like I'll never get up, Coach Powell, my daddy, the big, barrel-chested boys from the basketball team. I want them to feel better, but I can't make the words to tell them. I'm so confused.

The ambulance was going sixty-five when it hit me and now I'm bound to the bed at Baton Rouge General. My neck is broken, my spleen is gone, my lung is collapsed, and I'm not wearing any underwear. I don't know how long I've been here, but long enough that time has begun to take a new shape. Beyond the slivers of sunrise and darkness that sneak through the hospital shades, beyond the protocols and shifts and dosages and routines, I'm removed from the passing of hours, divorced from what was ordinary—cheerleading and algebra and Sunday dinner at my grandparents' house.

The doctors don't let me feel the pain. They keep it at a safe distance with a tingly calming medicine that goes through a needle in my hand and makes me sleep. The medicine doesn't let me feel anything at all. I notice the bumpy path of staples that leads up my belly from my pelvis to my sternum but I don't feel fear about them. I cry only once, when I find out they shaved the bottom of my head as bald as my daddy's. Everything my body is supposed to do is performed by someone or something else. A machine breathes for me; a long tube snakes down my windpipe to the edges of my lungs. The nurses thin my blood for me with little injections in my tummy. I'm a robot with skin.

The stream of visitors is constant, two at a time. They bring casseroles for my parents, black speckled lilies and tea roses, and lots of tears.

What's the problem? Why are you crying? Don't cry.

I want to tell them. But I can't. I try scrawling on the bed-sheets with my fingers but nobody really understands. My hands are stuck to the bed and my voice has been taken from me, but everyone I love is here. I feel so, so loved and so, so confused. I drift in and out of a haze, not knowing where I'm going, but feeling as though I have a very long journey ahead of me.

1

Different Kinds of Smart

I am awake but I keep my eyes closed, letting only the small-est bit of light slip in. There's just enough hot, heavy Louisiana breath coming through the window screen to fog up the pane with the promise of another hundred-degree afternoon. The bird dogs start in, barking at the chicken feathers floating in the air and running circles in the kennel, but I am only listening for the sound of her feet on the floor. The farmhouse groans as the humidity rises and the air conditioner sputters to life. Finally, I can hear her.

My mom pads barefoot across the hallway and the smells of face cream we can't afford and Community Coffee settle on top of me. Her shadow crosses the threshold and I peek quickly at her glossy red toenails. Even at five years old, I know that she is beau-tiful, painted just the way a Southern woman should be.

"Mornin', RuRu," she sings.

I'm sprawled belly down on a trundle bed between my big brothers, a lanky, big-eyed doll with salty morning breath. She

3

rubs up and down my back and scoops me up the way she always does, forearm in the crook of my knee, left shoulder a pillow for my cheek, and we walk. She knows I am awake, but she pretends so that I can, so that we can keep dancing our favorite dance.

Coffeepot steam and dust come to me in warm, sour clouds as we move down the stairs. I sniff hard and worry it will give me away. I am not ready to be done with our game yet and there are still a few more steps left to go, *creak, creak, creak*, down the stairs and past the kitchen.

Her feet sink into the plush rug and go quiet. We have arrived. She sets me in their bed next to the hearth that is my daddy. His big, warm body is a furnace you'd think I could never need in July, but that I cannot do without. I snuggle right into him.

"Pat, pat. Rub, rub," he coos as his hand sweetly finds the spot between my shoulders. "God loves you. Daddy loves you."

We wait together for a stretch of time that has never felt long enough. We wait until the bugs scream louder than the birds and the world comes calling for us. This is my most sacred space, where joy lives. This is where I begin.

St. Francisville is small, a half speck of a town. For a child, though, it is just the right size. In this place between the sticks and the swamp, joy is growing everywhere; it's always within arm's reach. You could hack away at it if you wanted to but it would always grow right back, bigger and fuller and wilder than it was before. Lots of things grow wild here. The live oaks are covered in mossy Muppet hair, palm leaves poke through the picket fences and tickle your legs when you walk, and love is the long, leathery vine that wraps itself around all of it. It's comically Southern, but I don't really know it yet. On Fridays, the boys play football and the girls wave cellophane pom-poms. On Saturdays, the women whisper about all of it, attaching scandal to every glance exchanged between daughters and sons. The men just smile and shake their heads. On Sundays we all slip into our church clothes and watch the hot sun shining in through the stained glass in Popsicle-colored laser beams. My daddy sits next to me in the pew and points out the dove in the stained-glass window.

"Every time you see the bird, know your daddy's thinking about you, that he loves you so much."

He snuggles me under his arm and I count the minutes until I get to ring the church bell, until my toes lift up off the ground from the weight of it and I feel like I'm flying, until my daddy walks me around and shows me off and I am delighted in by friends, strangers, and everyone in between.

Our little farm is only twenty minutes away from Grace Episcopal Church. We don't have much money or any neighbors I can play with, but I have space here to be whoever I want to be, a Rockette, a fairy godmother, LL Cool J. I am loved ferociously in whatever costume I put on. We have hundreds of acres of land that my grandfather passed down to us, thick forests where the long blacksnakes move and wide-open fields where the deer tiptoe stealthily in the morning. My tap shoes sound like gunfire in the quiet of the country as I dance across our big, wide porch in my bathing suit. I dance everywhere I go, shimmying my shoulders for strangers in the grocery store and kids on the playground, for anyone who will watch me. I like the way music moves me. I keep dancing until little pearls of wetness drip down the hollow of my back, until I'm sick and dizzy from cartwheels, until fatigue wraps me up in its arms and brings me in for dinner.

My daddy is the principal at Wilkinson County Christian Academy across the border in Woodville, Mississippi. I go to school there. He is beloved and respected and cherished by everyone, from the lunch ladies to the teenagers he busts for cutting class. They delight in him and he likes being delighted in just as much as I do. He wears a bow tie and a sport coat and glasses with perfectly circular frames. I think he looks dignified, like Colonel Sanders disguised as Sherlock Holmes, and I get the biggest rush of pride when I see him. The second the bell rings at 3 p.m., he transforms back into Daddy: he rolls up his sleeves and undoes his tie, and he giggles and bops with me the whole way up Highway 61. When we get home, he leaves me to go play in the earth like a little boy, plowing the garden with his mule, running his dogs, and feeding the horses sweet-smelling scoops of grain. Our farm is his favorite place in the whole world.

The dogs follow him everywhere, to Texas for quail season, to the porch to read a book, to the back field to be relieved from their suffering when they're old and sick. Vietnam follows him everywhere, too, but he tries never to look back at it; he never talks about it. Instead of remembering, he rebels against it with goodness. He shares vegetables from our garden and fish from our pond with his poor friends, and he does it with a graciousness that makes it seem as though they are rescuing us from our okra and watermelon. He tells us every day at breakfast, "I love you, remember your manners, always look out for the little guy." I want to be just like him. Every time my Timex flashes something special like 11:11 or 12:34, I make a wish, and it's always the same: *Make me be good, make me love Jesus, make me like Daddy.*

My middle brother, Tim, doesn't have to wish for my daddy's heart like I do—he has a heart like God's, sure and unspoiled. He's always sweeping porches, helping neighbors, and listening to the long, tiresome stories of people who have no one else to tell them to. He moves through his day quietly and thoughtfully, like a little granddad, and expects nothing in return for his goodness but for more people to experience God's unconditional love. It's infuriating. The grown-ups adore him. The first Sunday in December, my mom gives us dozens of pumpkin bread wrapped in tinfoil and ribbon to deliver to her friends in town. She gives me fifteen loaves to pass out but trusts Tim with just two, knowing he will spend hours sipping unsweet tea with the elderly, staring at their old photos, and holding on to each gnarled hand that greets him. He doesn't even like unsweet tea but he'd never trouble a person by asking for sugar.

My older brother, Lile, gets a mountain of pumpkin bread—it seems to grow every year—and we deliver it all together. He's different from Tim, his voice rings out loud and deep from his chest and he is almost always chased by the laughter of the sparkly-eyed high school girls who shadow him. He listens to Guns N' Roses and cusses and makes my daddy so angry he screams, but he can also be a teddy bear and I get to see his very softest side. He says that from the moment I came home from the hospital, I've been his. He would sit with me in his lap for an hour and just stroke my fat baby cheek while his friends ran amok outside in the yard. He's my protector, my safest place, and he lets me sleep in his room until he leaves to go to school at LSU in Baton Rouge.

I am the darling of our family, I know that. I am loved wholeheartedly and that's the way I learn to love people back. I'm a doter, a gusher, and every time I leave my parents, even if I'm just going out to play, I tell them, "Bye! I love you! You're my favorite, I'll never forget you!"

I don't know what hurt is until I'm six years old and in second grade. School is the first hurt, the one that makes shame creep up my throat and numb my lips. Nobody knows why I can't spell *animal* or *table*, why my brain can't seem to sit still even when my body does. The hot red rungs of the playground stare at me through the window every afternoon and warm my back when poor Miss Ashley is trying to teach me all the different types of clouds. An empty swing swinging or a Twinkie wrapper tumbling across the dirt are invitations to adventures that my imagination can't pass up. I get itchy, I squirm, I chatter. "Ruthie! Miss Lindsey!" they call, but nobody can reach me in the little white room.

Even though my daddy is my school's principal, he doesn't care that my brain is different. He speaks a different language of learning than most people do. He knows how to reach me wherever I am.

I'm eight years old when he teaches me about *Magnolia fuscata*. I'm sitting near the leaf of our dining table sticking pencil shavings into the crevice and trying to memorize the names of Louisiana's common trees and bushes. I study them hard in my science book, but they all look the same to me, shiny green images plopped down onto giant blocks of text. I read it over and over again, the information gets lost over and over again, everything in my brain gets scrambled. I cry and I wait for him.

"Come with me," he whispers, gliding up beside me from no-where and cupping his hand near my ear.

I look up at him, eyes halfway drowned, and he smiles at me. He takes my hand and we step out barefoot onto the thick green of the yard. The last strokes of pink stretch across the tree line. It's dusk; there's just enough light for our faces to glow.

"Take a deep breath, baby," he says.

I count aloud, "One, two, three," and have a big glug of the evening. He does it too. Then, he tells me the reasons the air smells like honey; he teaches me about all the good things that grow here.

"That's a silver bell," he says. The tree is gangly, with branches that shoot out from its middle and have more white flowers on them than leaves.

"This one's a coral honeysuckle."

He lifts a red, bugle-shaped cone to my face and I stick my nose into it. I expect sweetness but get pollen instead.

"It doesn't smell like much, does it?" He shrugs. "The hum-mingbirds sure love it though!"

He leads me through the yard, pointing at his favorites as I squeal with delight. We run our fingers through a carpet of blue phlox in the garden, we lean against the smooth cypress bark at the edge of the forest, and I stand up to my waist in irises. Then he shows me his favorite one of all.

"*Magnolia fuscata*."

He likes to use the fancy words for things when he can.

We run around to the side of the house. The smell of fresh banana bread travels through my nose and becomes syrup at the back of my throat. The tree is young and skinny, covered in green buds waiting to become yellow flowers. The smell is everywhere; I sway in it and hope it gets stuck in my hair. He plucks off a bud and sticks it up his nose. I laugh so hard at the ridiculous sight of him that I stumble and scare the lightning bugs, which have just flicked on at our ankles.

"Now that's what home smells like." He smiles, raising his eyebrows high above his glasses; he knows he's gotten me curious enough to try. I pluck two buds from the branch, wiggle them into my nostrils, and breathe the most delicious, unforgettable breaths of my life. We stand there doing nothing but breathing, giggling, and letting the smell of home sink to the deepest pockets of our bellies. I love him almost more than I can bear.

Magnolia fuscata. I put it in a part of my brain where I know I won't ever lose it.

My mom loves me differently than my daddy does. She thinks I'm the prettiest thing she's ever seen, even though I have giant hair and teeth like a donkey. She gussies me up in smocked dresses and big bows and shows me off wherever we go, twirling me around and bragging, "Ruthie makes friends wherever she goes. Her legs are longer than mine are."

It makes my cheeks flush. My mom is from the city; she was set up with my daddy by a friend, and when he called her, they found out that their apartments were in the exact same building. She was a flight attendant and he worked at something she calls a "fat cat" bar in the French Quarter. They got married and he moved her out to the country. The glamour of New Orleans followed her, and so did the gin-drunk ghost of her dad. Just like my daddy, though, she tries not to look back at the things that haunt her. Mom is elegant, whether she's brushing her teeth or baking a pie, and I feel clumsy and awkward when I stand beside her. She's a big black-eyed swan who somehow ended up with a pelican baby.

The summer before third grade, she takes me shopping for school supplies at the Walgreens one town over, in Zachary. We go for frozen yogurt after, even though it's only ten-thirty in the morning, and this is where I learn about different types of smart.

We are the first people through the door, and inside the air of the TCBY is so cold I get goose bumps on my arms. My mom waits for me in a little booth while I order; she doesn't want anything, she's only eating grapefruit right now. The girl behind the counter heaps Oreo crumble on top of my cup and smiles at me. She has a tiny stud in her nose and pink hair and I like her right away. Even though I am young, I know that it isn't easy to be different here and I know that she is brave. I smile back at her as big as I can; she adds an extra scoop of black cookie dust and winks at me. I carry the heaping cup of yogurt across the room, plonk it down on the table, and nudge an extra spoon toward my mom. She grins, takes a few bites, and tells me I'm naughty.

"Baby," she explains, lifting a big eyebrow, "there are different kinds of smart. Some people, like your daddy, are smart with books. . . ."

She continues explaining that there are all types of things people can be good at and I try to pay attention while the vanilla melts on my tongue. All I can think about is how pretty she is, hair swept over one eye like an exotic movie star who smokes cigarettes and drives on the wrong side of the road. She touches my arm to bring me back to her, bubble-gum-pink cheeks falling into perfect shadow valleys above her jaw.

"Ru, you are smart with people. Being people smart is a beautiful gift you have; everyone loves you because you know how to love them so well. I wish I had it when I was a young woman."

None of it makes sense to me. I feel the yogurt dribbling down my chin onto the collar of the denim jacket she begged me not to wear and I wonder why she would want to be anything like me. She looks a little sad, she does that sometimes, but I don't really understand why.

The electronic doorbell sounds as a pregnant lady shoves her sweaty shoulder into the glass. I jump up and hold it open for her, cooled air forming a smile on her face as she waddles inside. I tell her she looks pretty and she beams at me. My mother is right, I am people smart.

The yogurt turns to slop and I pitch it in the garbage can. I wave to the pregnant lady and the girl behind the counter and we leave.

When class begins that August, school becomes a place of learning again, because school is where I work on my people smarts. People need different things from me: this is my first lesson. Some people need a comedian who blows bubbles in her chocolate milk, others need a big sister to ward off bullies. Lots of people just need a safe place to stash their secrets, and though I can hardly ever keep them, they tell me anyway. I learn that almost all people need to feel like they belong to someone, so I let them know that they are important to me. By October I find myself belonging to nearly everyone: the basketball kids, the Bible study kids, even the teachers who wonder if they should really be telling a girl who still plays with Barbies about their husband's "friend" Rita from work who is only twenty-nine years old. My mom is so proud of me for fitting in that she could bust.

My second lesson is in performing, summoning any version of myself that a person might like to be around. In between classes, I sit in a bathroom stall and wait, listening to the high school gossip about who is on their period, who got the water-filled bra from the Victoria's Secret in Baton Rouge, and who is in love with Lile. When the last pair of sneakers has squeaked across the floor, I find my way to the mirror and try to be all the different things I've seen in people before. I try to be shy like Marlene Peek, the mysterious and beautiful girl in class. I try to be sexy like Cindy Crawford; I pull up my shirt and suck my belly deep into my ribs until my body looks like the number eight. I give up after just a minute, puff my tummy out, and do a silly dance. I'm really not any good at pretending to be someone else. What I *am* good at is smiling. Smiling is my third lesson—it can help you belong to just about anyone. I stretch my mouth so far that I can count seventeen teeth in the mirror and my eyes almost disappear into my cheeks.

How to belong changes with time and I don't like it. One day in sixth grade a skirt gets folded over at the waist, the next day thirty skirts follow. Strawberry ChapStick becomes Revlon in colors called Toast of New York and Champagne on Ice, the girls become young women. The boys remain boys, but my friends begin to picture them as men; a few even declare to them that they are "boyfriends," though a relationship born on Monday rarely lasts through lunch on Wednesday. The changes are scary. I have no desire to kiss a forty-eight-hour boyfriend or spend twenty minutes in the shower trying to shave the sable hair off my legs. I still want to play with dolls and get tucked in at night. Without the belonging, though, without my people smarts, I don't know who I am. It makes people happy when I pretend and the pink lipstick looks pretty on me.

My mother loves the changes that have come with twelve. I am orbiting another inch closer to her than I was at eleven and it thrills her. My friend Susan's birthday is just two days before mine, and to celebrate, our moms take us clothes shopping in New Orleans, where we stick our toes into womanhood. They drink orange juice and sparkling wine at lunch and let us order Shirley Temples and virgin daiquiris, though neither Susan nor I have any idea what a virgin or a daiquiri actually is. It all feels very important and grown-up, soaking our skin in the sun and stumbling sober over the cobblestones, but when the conversations about clothes and boys begin, I wander away the same way I do in social studies, back to the hot red rungs of the playground. Susan's mind does not wander. The next phase of life has summoned her and she has arrived with wobbly wedge sandals and choker necklaces and CK One perfume that smells like the ocean. I'm just not ready. I plod along beside her with my shopping bag, terrified of being left behind.

After we return from the city, my daddy lets Susan and me drive his busted old truck over the cattle gap and down the dirt lane that leads from our little farmhouse to the road. We pull ourselves up onto the squishy vinyl seats and knot our shirts above our navels.

"Are you serious?!" Susan squeals when I turn the ignition. They don't let kids drive much in the suburbs.

For her, stuck in the middle of town, bound by the rules of town living, it is the ultimate liberation. As she grins at me, two rows of braces gleaming, I understand that I belong to Susan and I understand who she needs me to be: an accomplice, a sister, a fellow traveler on the journey to thirteen. So I smile big like I always do. When I smile big, people like me, and even if I'm uncomfortable, I want to be liked. I join Susan, meet her and the other girls on the precipice of womanhood. It's the last place I want to be. I'd rather be at home playing with dolls than trying to become one.

Black smoke flies from the tailpipe, making chemical waves in the air as we *chug, chug, chug* along, home and my daddy and twelve years old getting smaller behind us. Susan's family owns a grocery store and she has brought us six plastic bottles of root beer in her backpack; we swig and cheers with them like beers as our bony bottoms bounce up and down, voices rattling through "Knockin' Boots" by Candyman. We throw our heads back and cackle, candy cigarettes in hand, at the imaginary herd of teenage boys chasing behind. Of course, they want to make out with us. The idea of wet lips pressing up against mine makes me feel seasick and panicked. I can't even say the word *sex* above a whisper, and every time I see a pregnant lady I blush, knowing exactly what she did to become that way. I don't want to grow up but Susan does and the other girls do. I play along, smile big, and keep my youngness a secret. The lustful, make-believe boys chase us until the afternoon sinks into the ground. We don't know it yet, but it will only be a couple of years before our silly game becomes real.

"GO FASTER," Susan begs.

The truck lurches forward, soda splashes on our jean shorts, and she squeals, taking a long drag of her "Camel." All I can think about is how happy she is, how she feels alive and loved with me. I wag a finger at the phantom suitors behind us and she almost doubles over.

"Ruthie!" she howls as we rumble along.

I am people smart, I tell myself again.

At the end of the day, when the edges of the earth turn Sunkist orange, Susan goes back to her house in Woodville and I sit alone in the hot, rubbery bucket of the truck drinking piss-warm root beer and smoking a stick made of sugar. The farther I grow from the ground, the more years I build on to my life, the more I will catch myself thinking about this place and this time, a time where I get swept up in the colors of the sky and where I burst into song and dance for reasons I can't ever pin down. This is where I begin.

2

Black & White

She tells me at the Egg Roll King over shiny tan dumplings and Szechuan chicken.

"We'll get to vacation *all over* the country!"

My mom's lashes are pulled all the way up, big velvet curtains hanging over her pretty eyes.

"California! Miami! New York!" she says, making a list for herself. She stuffs her sandals into an imaginary suitcase and wets her lips.

We're sitting in our booth, the one we always sit in, right near the door, where our faces glow peach and blue from the neon of the OPEN sign. People go by, mostly middle-aged ladies, and they peer in at the sweet mother-daughter window display we make for them. We both like the way it feels when they look at us.

Egg Roll King is my mother's favorite place to eat, even though it is cheap and dirty. The dining room looks more like a basement than a restaurant; shiny wood panels with big brown knots stretch all the way from the black grout to the splotchy ceiling. The calendar that hangs near the register is stuck on May 1988, which was almost five years ago. There are no proper linens, no flowers in the ladies' room, and no garden salads on the menu, but it is our place and nobody else knows about it. I love coming here with my mom. She shovels hunks of shimmering pink pork into her mouth without counting Weight Watchers points, welcomes the smell of Clorox and peanut oil into her clothing, and makes friends with all the waiters. It isn't a place to be seen—none of her friends are about to pop through the door, so she can relax. I can relax too.

I thought we were here to celebrate. I made the cheerleading squad and even though nearly everyone does, my parents decided to be proud of me. I decided to let them. We eat appetizers, make small talk, and then she reaches around four bright bowls of sauce to grab my hands.

"Ruthie, I have some news."

My father has accepted a job as the superintendent of West Feliciana Parish and I have to go to a new school. It's a big deal for him, a promotion, an opportunity, a raise in pay, an honor, even. For me, it's a disaster. I slump down deep into the squeaky vinyl while she tries to get me excited: I'll get a VW convertible bug when I turn sixteen, just like the blue one that she had, we'll go shopping at the Ralph Lauren outlet, I can get highlights in my hair.

"Ru." She smiles. "You'll get to go to a new high school."

"A new high school?"

I want to seek shelter from the words the second I say them out loud.

High school.

I am thirteen years old. I haven't even gotten my period yet. I am six feet tall and barely a hundred pounds. I wear plastic-rimmed glasses, and they don't make me look smarter. My boy body hasn't even considered changing yet and I don't really want it to. WCCA is my second home. West Feliciana High is a whole different planet, a planet populated exclusively by teenage strangers doing strange teenage things. I'm not ready.

Perfectly manufactured plans for our future are still popping out of my mom's conveyor-belt mouth when the waiter arrives with the bill and two fortune cookies wrapped in crinkly plastic. I smash mine with my palm and pull a long slip of paper out of the crumbs:

LIFE IS FULL OF CHANGES. STAY FLEXIBLE.

I ball it up between my fingers and toss it on the table.

The first week of July, my mother secures us an invite to a swimming party at her friend Miss Patty's house. Miss Patty has a pool shaped like an enormous jellybean and a propane grill with seventeen knobs built right into the patio. She and the other moms organized this so that all the daughters going to West Feliciana High could get to know each other and so that they themselves could drink chardonnay in the afternoon. Miss Patty doesn't have a daughter my age, but in St. Francisville all the children belong to all the grown-ups, so it doesn't really matter.

Well-fed wasps fly in endless circles over plastic pitchers of lemonade and open bags of Cheetos when we arrive, and they greet us with their lazy, staticky bug buzz. I can hardly see anything over the giant, sweaty stacks of cut-up watermelon we've brought with us, but I hear Miss Patty's sugary voice and follow it to a sturdy, manicured hedge that she's using as a tabletop for her wine. She gives my mom and me each a wiggly hug and a ten-second biography of every girl in attendance.

There are a dozen girls sprawled all over with lemon-juice blond streaks in their hair and the brown, freckle-free skin of summer. About half have free-fallen into adolescence, having woken up one morning with breasts the size of hamburger buns, meaty thighs, and the good sense to put on a bikini; the rest wait impatiently on the trusses of that same bridge for their turn to jump, bodies stretched out and skinny, with empty triangular flaps of Lycra on their chests. I know that I'm different from them right away. Nobody is splashing or playing; they're just hot dogs on lounge chairs, grilling in the heat, talking about boys and haircuts. If this is puberty, I volunteer to leap last.

"Are you ready?" my mom asks. She and Miss Patty have been busy unloading the latest gossip from town.

I swallow and nod, and they leave me to join the other ladies under the swirling fan on the porch.

I lay my faded flower-print towel on a chair, pull my swimsuit from my butt, and walk toward the poolside.

The first girl I meet is called Andrea, and she is best friends with Lori. The next one I meet looks old enough to be a dental hygienist; she is best friends with Traci, who used to be best friends with a girl named Amy, who wasn't even invited to this party. The entire yard is filled with pairs, chosen sisters who will display their firmly cemented alliances in the new hallways come August. I think about my sweet Christian school where everybody was invited to everything, where everyone got to belong. My chest starts to ache as they gab about French-tip nails and crushes. I've been special plenty of times but never "different," and I'm surprised by how empty it feels. I stick my feet into the bathwater of the pool and wait for the day to be over and then for the school year to begin.

I am one of the youngest students at West Feliciana High, and though there is no uniform, I wear Bermuda shorts and a polo shirt on my first day because that's what I've always worn to school. My daddy kisses me on the head before I go in. He is wearing his uniform too: a bow tie, a tweed jacket, a sturdy Swiss army watch, and a little bit of breakfast on his shirt.

"You're going to do great. Everyone will love you."

He says this to both of us with complete confidence and I try my best to believe in me the way that he does. I push open the big doors and prepare myself to feel the feeling I had at Miss Patty's, my differentness.

A few lockers down from mine, a pregnant girl balances a brown-bagged lunch on her belly and boys disguised as men walk around in clouds of ashtray smell. There are girls with coasters stuck into their earlobes and hair as shockingly blue as the lunch trays. It is the busiest place I have ever been. The first week, I bob along in the fast-moving stream of students, electrically charged from listening to sixteen conversations at once, from walking into whooshes of drugstore cologne. There is differentness everywhere and nobody seems to care much about it, or to notice, really. Just in case my differentness starts to feel heavy again, I go to the place where I know I belong, where all girls above six feet tall are welcome: the basketball team.

Different isn't bad, but different can be complicated, it can be painful, it can even be scary. When I walk into the gym, shorts

21

sliding down the knobs of my hips, sniffing desperately for the familiar smells of new shoes and the floor wax that makes everything so shiny, I realize that I'm the only white girl on the team. At the time, there were only a handful of black kids at my old school. WCCA began as a segregation academy in the late 1960s, and even when the doors were open to everyone back then, not many students of color seemed to want to walk through them, understandably. Most of the black people I've ever met have been in service.

In St. Francisville, the white people live in the nice neighborhoods and many of the black people live in Hardwood: This is how it has always been. Hardwood is an area stuck right in the middle of town, with clusters of low apartment buildings and parched brown grass. It's a bit of an island, nothing but highway and straw-colored fields on either side. The streets are called A, B, C, D, like they couldn't decide on proper names and just gave up. White people don't hang out there. We drove through only one time, to drop up off a man my daddy picked up on the side of the road. Sleek shorthaired dogs with dangly nipples belonging to no one and everyone at the same time trot along the sidewalk, music heartbeats out of open windows, and children play in the rippling, corduroy heat without the cover of trees to shade them. I don't know why there is separateness, only that it's existed much longer than I have, before this town had a name. Even my daddy, a champion of all people, stays politely behind the invisible lines that history drew.

Today, the gym is cold. The air-conditioning is working overtime to catch up with the end-of-summer heat. Goose bumps rise all at once on my skin. The girls stop bouncing their balls, smacking rubber against parquet, when they see me coming toward them. I walk, chalky, straw-shaped legs; clumsy, skinny hips; differentness on full display. I wonder if this is how they feel at the good grocery store or at the wrong church. I keep walking toward the center circle in my too-big shorts.

"Hi! I'm Ruthie!"

Before I can say anything else, they wrap my plywood-stiff body into the biggest, warmest hug, and I wonder if maybe differentness doesn't have to be complicated at all. Maybe it never had to be?

Five nights a week under the fire-bright lights, I come alive. My basketball girls, Frannie, the two Pams, and Jamise, love me without hesitation, without judgment, and without the slightest bit of disdain for me never asking the questions that my parents never asked either. I become the closest with Frannie; she is an entire foot too short to play, so she takes statistics for the team instead. We have nothing in common besides the freckles on our noses, but we love each other completely. She likes Cat Stevens and I like Snoop Dogg; she's quiet and serene and I'm too loud nearly everywhere we go. The grown-ups look at us a little funny when we're out together, but we don't care. Frannie welcomes me into her world fully and fearlessly, even though she has never truly been welcomed in mine. I visit her church, where the service seems to last all day long, and I sit out in the sun and smoke of Hardwood, drinking in the sweetness of neighbors who pass out paper plates of food so full that they buckle at the middle. After we eat, we lie on the dead grass with Frannie's little cousins cuddled up next to us looking up at the fluffy plumes of grill smoke rising to the sky. I think about the girls who were supposed to become my friends sprawled out on lounge chairs at the pool party. None of them were black. At those kinds of parties, they never are.

My time in high school melts fast, like butter in a microwave. I sit at a different table every day in the cafeteria and make friends with anyone who will let me set my lunch tray beside theirs, no matter what they look like. I stop pining for the smallness and sameness of my little Christian school in Mississippi. I like the way the borders of my world have dissolved. The kids at West Feliciana, kids of all colors studying together and playing ball together, seem to have figured something out that no one else has yet beyond the brown-brick campus. As I drive home every afternoon to the smallness and sameness of St. Francisville, I begin to ask myself the questions that nobody asks out loud:

Why don't you let your daughters date black boys?

Why aren't we supposed to be friends outside of school?

Why are you looking at my friend that way when she shops at your store?

Why does different have to be so complicated here?

I begin to want answers.

It is senior year and we are still in the hot, sticky part of fall just before October. There is a white dance at Grace Episcopal and I invite my black friends to come with me. White dances have been happening in St. Francisville since before I was born. No one would ever call them "white dances" of course, but the black kids are never invited, they are never missed. The dances are organized by the Ladies in Pearls, an informal mishmash guild of big-haired and breathy-voiced white women who are always walking quickly and dressed for brunch. I've been taught to respect my elders, it's one of the most important rules in our house, so I work hard to impress them. They organize everything in St. Francisville, from the Mardi Gras parade to the monthly bingo game at the senior center. They do lots of good, spending days before Christmas mashing potatoes and basting big bronze turkeys to feed the homeless, praying for anyone who will let them, and working tirelessly to keep the smell of fresh honeysuckle pumping through town like casino oxygen. But most of them don't even know where Hardwood is.

There are six of us that night. We crank forward the seat of my friend Kendrick's two-door Toyota and collapse into a Polo-perfumed pile of legs and hands that linger on top of each other. The sky has just gotten dark; a gauzy thicket of starlight stretches all around us as the car bumps along Royal Street to Jackson Hall, a church event venue just far enough out of God's peripheral vision for weddings and parties to get out of hand. We park near the old cemetery and I look out at big old Grace Church spouting up out of the ground and towering above the mossy concrete slabs and I think about the perfect white dove in the stained-glass window. I know what we're doing is right. There are quiet hymns coming from somewhere, maybe from Grace, maybe from the Catholic church next door, or the Baptist church a few streets over, the long mournful calls for Jesus mixing awkwardly with the *ka-thud* of the speakers from Jackson Hall, sacred Confederate-era grounds now rumbling with Warren G and Blackstreet. None of us catch the irony; we just like the "No Diggity" song.

The Ladies in Pearls stand just inside the door, assembled in a floral polyester barricade. Their eyes travel slowly over the group of us, taking in the dark skin and sparrow-brown eyes from behind the safety of their folding table. They frown.

"What can we do for you tonight, Ruthie?"

The head of the PTA, Miss Charlotte, purses her pink-lined lips and stretches them out into a squeaky, patent-leather grin.

"We'd like six tickets, please, ma'am."

She drums her nails across the tin cashbox, trying to decide where she stands on the issue standing in front of her.

Jamise, the cocaptain of the cheerleading team, tugs at my belt loop. "Let's just go, Ru."

I look back at my friends' faces, etched with disappointment, fear, and sadness. The next rap song in the queue begins to play while the Ladies in Pearls mull over whether they should let black kids into a white dance playing only black music. I can't take it anymore.

I slap sixty dollars on the table.

"Six tickets, please."

I grab a whole ribbon of them from Miss Charlotte and push past her, not waiting for permission. We dance for hours, until the lights flicker on, hoping that maybe they'll see that different doesn't have to be complicated anymore.

The Ladies are still behind their table when we leave; we say "Thank you" because it's a reflex and walk down the steps. The sound of my name bounces off the bricks to my ears and I know they're talking about me, "Lloyd's girl." Jamise hears it too. She links her arm through mine and walks me away while my jaw shakes. I feel shame. I know that I don't deserve to be in trouble but I am. I try to shake off the feeling at the after-party.

The old ranch bungalow stretches half the length of the street and sits on top of a big slope of grass. A junior named Charlie lives here. Rusty patio furniture is scattered across the lawn and the lighter fluid stink of a two-story bonfire is almost enough to mask the skunky smell of weed being packed into pretty glass pipes. We scatter when we get here: Kendrick goes to help pick the music, Jamise finds the other cheerleaders, and I find Brian, who is my favorite person to flirt with and be next to. I go out back and plop down onto his lap while the volleyball team drinks cheap, candy-flavored wine and gossips. I laugh along with them and pretend that they're hilarious, because I can't stop thinking about Jackson Hall, because I want to feel like I belong again. An hour passes quickly. I watch them get drunker and sillier and I let Brian rub the lowest part of my back all the way to the frilly top borders of my underwear.

People begin to pair off and make out with each other, and though Brian looks at me with hopeful puppy-dog eyes, I go out front to find my friends. I search inside the house and by the fire but I can't find them anywhere. Our parking spot is empty. A group of boys from the baseball team pull me behind a fat magnolia tree and point toward the porch. Charlie's mother is standing there, arms crossed, cordless phone tucked into her waistband like a pistol. She asked my friends to leave, which we all knew was because they were black. The baseball boys shake their heads and shrug their shoulders when they tell me, like there's nothing in the world we can do about it. I know that I should leave, we all should, but none of us want to be the one to stir the pot that's been boiling for more than a century. I stay at the party. I eat the pizza that Charlie's mom bought for us and I laugh and dance while somewhere in town, Jamise and the rest of my friends look for a place they're allowed to be. I play innocent bystander just like the rest, because I'm afraid, because I'm still trying to impress the grown-ups, even though I'm practically grown myself. We all pretend to be innocent, but none of us are.

At school Brian will tell me that the Ladies at Jackson Hall were calling me names. I refuse to print those words, I refuse to dignify them as language. It breaks my heart when I hear them. I know that the Ladies are wrong, they're afraid, they're awful, but still I feel shame. Jamise and Kendrick never bring up what happened and I don't either. They don't call me coward or ask me why I stayed; they continue to love and accept me, performing a deeper, more profound act of grace than I can comprehend at sixteen years old. We keep our friendship stowed safely inside the walls of the big brown school for now, only letting it sun itself on the dried-out lawns of Hardwood.

We don't know it yet, but soon our friendship will move to another big brown building a few towns away, and everything that stands between our worlds, the differentness, won't matter anymore.

3

Always Go Left

The tiny maroon 1988 Honda Accord I drive used to be Lile's. It has the friendly headlights that pop out of the hood when the roads go dark and make it look silly, like a cartoon robot. Lile decided "it" was a "she" as soon as he turned the key in the ignition. He drove her to football games and backfield parties and to pick up his very first date. When I turned sixteen, he came home, handed me the keys, and taught me to drive stick. He clung patiently to the door handle as I jostled him up and down the driveway and through the fields, stomping on the clutch, yanking the gearshift, and making a mess of the gravel. The troubling moans that rumbled from the gearbox couldn't have been easy for him to ignore, but he did so anyway, grinning over every bump, through every lurch. The Accord is a family heirloom, no different than a grandma's wedding ring or pocket watch, and I am honored when the keys are passed down to me—even though the insides stink so badly of sweaty football gear and Old Spice, I check under the seat for a pair of socks every so often just to be sure. The only thing that doesn't work close to perfectly is the CD player, but I keep trying it anyway. Driving without music feels as strange as dancing without it.

Today I'm going to Baton Rouge with my friends; there are four carfuls of us. We're stopped outside the little store at the gas station where the old man sells big plastic bottles of vodka and cans of Miller Lite to anyone with a wallet. The place is built entirely of tin and changes hands so frequently that they don't even bother with a sign anymore. The lights from Jetson Juvenile Corrections Center are so close they practically shine into the lot, but nobody seems too worried about getting caught. Brian and I are the only ones who don't drink, so we wait in the car and talk about the trip. We're almost halfway to the Hooters in Baton Rouge; we're stopping there for wings before continuing on to Celebration Station, a carnival that never shuts off. It has hot dogs and arcade games and a track of sluggish go-karts that are slower than my daddy's riding mower. It's supposed to be "Fun for the Whole Family," but at night it's mostly just teenagers like us who want to make out in secret behind the batting cages and put their sticky, funnel cake–slick hands all over each other. Even though I'm not ready to date yet, I like watching the way the boys and girls perform there. The boyfriends pump all their quarters into the machine with the bionic, toy-grabbing hand while the girlfriends look on, pretending that they can't live without a plush panda bear. The boyfriends are always disappointed to learn that one unit of teddy bear is not equal in value to a hand job behind the big resin mountain on the putt-putt course.

I can see our friends inside the gas station through the smeary window, the girls riding piggyback on the boys through the aisles, cruising slowly past the ice chest and learning about alcohol as they go. Next to the grown-up bottles of white wine and the copper-colored liquors called Jack Daniel's and Captain Morgan, they look younger and more nervous than they actually are. Brian smiles at me from across the car, rolling his Neptune-blue eyes at the others for taking too long and stretching his arms back behind his head. He is wearing businessman clothes today, snow-white button-down shirt pulled out from his khaki pants and sleeves rolled all the way up to his elbows. He looks handsome but I decide not to tell him; I just look over and giggle while he tries to unbutton his collar. I hate dressing up. I don't think Brian likes it much either.

"I was just at a party for my grandpa." He shrugs. His cheeks go pink and shiny and it makes me giggle harder. I grab a CD to fiddle with before I start to turn pink too. It's a local rapper's CD that somebody gave me. It's been lent to at least five people in school and has finally made its way to me. I push it into the groaning dash. The stereo gums it for a minute and spits it back out.

"Ruuuuthie," Brian says. He's seen me try a hundred times before.

The square-shaped letters march across the screen, "C-A-N-N-O-T R-E-A-D," and I make my sad face for him, the one I know that he melts for. He deposits a handful of my favorite soft peppermints, still warm from his pocket, into the cup holder. Brian has been doing a terrible job of keeping the secret that he loves me.

The doorbell from the shop slurs its battery-hungry song, *ding-dong, diiiiaaaang-dooooong*, and trails off as the kids who make up our caravan spring from the tin shack into the perfect fall night. Their shoes kick up gravel as they run across the lot waving their paper-bagged treasures in the air like we won't believe what's inside. This is what I always hoped seventeen years old would be: road trips and cheerleading and people drinking Smirnoff Ice. A boy named Jerome flashes his nipples at Brian as he runs past the car. I honk the horn at him and its sad lamb bleat makes all of us roar. Brian shakes his head and can't stop giggling. I could eat up every last crumb of senior year.

Our fleet of borrowed and inherited cars chugs to life. The gravel pops like corn kernels under the car tires as they all roll to the blacktop, pulling into a neat line at the edge of the road and waiting for the traffic to clear. Someone is listening to the Fugees so loud it makes the peppermints Brian brought rattle like dice. I put the car in reverse and try the CD player again just one more time, wiping the shiny tree-stump rings of the disc against my jeans. Brian throws his hands up in the air, the stereo slurps it up, sighs, and spits it out at us again.

"Ruthie, we gotta go," Brian says. I give in and let up on the brake.

Truck tires screech out onto the highway in front of us and send puffs of glimmering white dust into the air. They sparkle under the skyscraper-high lamps; we sit and watch it settle. It's the closest thing to snowfall in Louisiana. When it disappears, everyone is gone and I panic. I'm the last to leave and I don't know which way to go.

Later, when I become a woman, I'll be famous for my horrible sense of direction. I'll go to the wrong addresses and knock on the wrong doors, I'll get lost at Hartsfield-Jackson Airport in Atlanta and, in New York, I'll take the subway to Queens when I'm trying to go to Brooklyn. My friend Garrett will say that my instincts are so bad that I should always go left when my brain says to go right. At seventeen, years before GPS, MapQuest, and smartphones, I'm as good as lost if I can't keep up. So I just go. I surge ahead to find someone to follow and take a fast left. I forget to look as I cross over two lanes of traffic.

My body knows to scream before it even sees what is happening.

"Oh SHIT!"

My voice is echoey in the stillness. I see lights, big ones, slow comets swept down from the sky. The time moves drop by drop by drop from its faucet as the lights move closer, closer, closer. There is nothing we can do, we have only one second, two maybe. We sit, I smell the old football gear smell, Brian's shadow gets darker. We just wait together in the glow for what's about to happen to us.

An EMS Suburban slams into us going sixty-five miles per hour. It crunches my driver's-side door all the way across the car until it pokes out of the passenger window and flicks the car into a ditch.

Brian is still conscious when it's over, but I'm not. I abandon him in the fever dream and he has to navigate it all alone. He stares at me, hunched over the steering wheel. I'm silent for a few minutes and then my body gurgles back to life. I make strange raspy breathing sounds and Brian reaches for my hand. He says my name. For a while, it's all he says.

"Ruthie, Ruthie, Ruthie, Ruthie, Ruthie. Ruthie, Ruthie, Ruthie, Ruthie, Ruthie."

I don't respond, I just keep making my noises. He knows not to move me because he watches a lot of prime-time TV and there are car accidents on *Law & Order* all the time. He squeezes my hand, opens his car door, and stands on the side of the highway waving his hands, landing an airplane only he can see.

"Somebody! Help!"

"Call 911!"

People do stop, but Brian keeps yelling. He can't stop, there's nothing else to do with all the awful energy.

The driver of the Suburban is called Tony or Terry, he's a paramedic, and, like Brian, he's unharmed. Little glass nuggets that shine like diamonds crunch under his feet as he dodges the greasy, rainbow coolant puddles on the road that lead to me. He tells Brian to stay calm, that the ambulance is coming. They wait together and peer in at me through the windshield under a big round, bored moon that has seen everything before.

Wild red party lights come screaming up the highway ten minutes later and a team of men in navy-blue cargo pants pops out of the back. It is no Celebration Station, but it's definitely a carnival. For me, everything is muted, but sometimes I get a glimpse of the chaos. I'm glad I don't get more. They rush at me in the Accord—she's been pulverized into a grape-colored boomerang—and they whiz past Brian. They don't ask him if he's all right, they don't shine a little light in his eyes to make sure his pupils dilate properly, they just want to get me out.

On the outside, I am pristine, there is no rush of blood, no bones cranked into backward positions, not even a teardrop. I'm slumped over the steering wheel in the top corner of the car looking peaceful with my eyes shut. Brian can tell there's something wrong, though, something he can't see. They stabilize my neck and pull me out of the passenger door, unfolding me carefully like an instruction book and laying me out on a big red surfboard. Brian asks if I'm okay, but they don't answer.

People gather in the parking lot, on the roadside, and I come back for a moment. I can feel the surfboard moving under me and feel a face close to my face, hot breath and beard and serious eyes.

"*Hiss, hiss, hiss,*" I breathe at the face. It tells me to slow down.

With a *one, two, three*, I'm hoisted high and placed into the back of an ambulance. Brian is allowed to come with me into the boxy brightness and he sits as close as they'll let him. He asks if I'm going to be okay again, but they still won't answer. He decides to pray even though he's not religious and probably doesn't know if he's doing it right.

While he is busy talking to God, the ambulance rumbles down the road. A pair of slender scissors slip under my tank top and slide slowly up my navel to the middle of my bra. They slice right through it.

"Don't! Please don't! I don't want him to see me!"

It's too late. My nakedness wakes me up more.

I don't want him to see me. Not yet. I'm not ready.

Everything falls away from me, and my pale, never-seen breasts meet the cool air. I think about how naked I am while Brian prays and the men work. My mind stops remembering. I fall back asleep as my insides spill into each other, ruptured spleen bleeding inside me, punctured lungs purring under fractured ribs, neck broken.

I'm alive. If I had been hit by anyone else but a first responder, someone who knew not to move me, who knew I needed to be stabilized, I could be dead.

My mom is tossing a salad at her supper club in St. Francisville when she finds out. My daddy is just one room over drinking gin and tonics and telling jokes. It's November 2, his birthday; he's still full from the chocolate pie we ate in the afternoon and he's not sure he'll fit into the new clothes we got him from his Filson catalogue. He's peaceful when the police call with the news but he's not sure why.

"Marsha, Ruthie was in a wreck," he tells my mom calmly. "Everything is going to be okay."

Her arms drop to her sides; they're so heavy she can barely lift them. Mr. Carter, my godfather, leads them to his car. The hospital calls him on his boxy car phone and tells him I might be paralyzed. He prays while he drives. I have a 5 percent chance of survival and a 1 percent chance of walking again.

Tim is at our farmhouse doting on beautiful blond-haired Laura, his first girlfriend, whom we're all absolutely certain he will marry. They walk in the door from a trip to New Orleans and see the red square on the answering machine blinking frantically. He presses the button and before the message is complete, they get into the car. Lile is getting drunk and grilling meat at our hunting camp on the grassy fringes of Lake Rosemound just a few minutes from home. He does it every year with his work friends from Fred's Bar near LSU. My daddy sends two policemen for him since he knows they've been drinking Michelob since morning and nobody can drive. The cruiser bumps along the dirt path and scares the shit out of everyone when it gets there. As soon as they say my name, Lile jumps into the back seat, where they put the hoodlums, and begs the officers for more information. They don't have any, so they talk about their deer stands and wives instead while he falls to pieces behind the cage. They drop him at the local station and another unaffected cop takes him the rest of the way to me.

I wait for everyone at the hospital in Baton Rouge woozy and drunk on the strongest medicine.

"Excuse me, I'm very uncomfortable," I say as they send me through the MRI machine. They give me more medicine so I won't try to talk anymore. They tie my long arms and legs down with buckles because I don't want to be still.

My parents arrive just in time to see me. I'm shaking.

"Daddy, I don't think I can play basketball."

They roll me back under the big white movie-set lights to open my body and try to fix the mess inside. Lile won't get to talk to me before I go in but once he does arrive, he refuses to leave. He sleeps at a little desk in the waiting room with his head on a stack of phone books.

Exactly three weeks before, I am under another set of big white lights. It's halftime and I am waiting to find out if I'm homecoming queen. I change out of my cheerleading uniform, skirt cut extra long just for me, and into an ugly brown suit with too-short sleeves; they make all the girls wear them and none of us knows why. I walk out onto the field and stand beside my daddy. He tells me I look beautiful even though I'm dressed like an accountant and he makes a smile so big it wants to jump off his face. He knows I'm going to win. My mom watches on the sidelines in her cashmere sweater with tears beading at the edges of her eyes. In watching these milestones, she is completed in me, her only girl. She joyfully claims a part of the crown that they are about to balance on my frizzy hair, erasing a few stills of her own childhood and replacing them with this. It will leave a green smear on my forehead. My name sizzles out of the speakers and shocks me; I cup my hands over my mouth and double over the way they do on

TV, humbled and floored and surprised. Ten pounds of swaddled roses are placed gently into my arms; I cradle them and stroke the long dragon tails of greenery that poke out past the paper while the band plays a song that sounds very old. The whole town has shown up for me: they cheer for me and wave at me, blue-and-white foam fingers flapping under slow-falling confetti from God knows where. I'm unfolding exactly the way I'm supposed to. I wake up the next morning from the summit of high school expecting to feel transformed, expecting that the sweet-smelling flowers and the noise of my own name, the utter, quantifiable adoration I earned will have delivered me to a more complete love, but they haven't. It's all the same feelings, with a silver-plated crown on top.

When I wake up in Baton Rouge after the accident with a tube in my throat to help me breathe and my eyes burning, I will begin to learn. I will learn that love is not always a loud parade of a thing; it can be strong and silent. It is not the throb of my name across a football field but the low, tender call for me across a sterile room, a call from a person who knows they may never be heard but chooses to speak anyway. It is not the presentation of shiny crowns and shiny roses. It is the table filled with wrinkled petals and dirty water, the flowers that people brought not knowing if I would ever wake to see them. It is not sitting on the sidelines in a nice sweater watching me blossom, it is sitting by my bedside disheveled and barefaced, watching me wither. I will learn that love is one person becoming undone for another. It's being stripped of the protective armor we've worked hard to fashion for ourselves to become the armor for somebody else. It's standing naked and shivering before what scares us the most to honor what it is that we love the most. This is the love that will transform me.

4

Chuncky and
My Other Best Friends

I open my hands to them. Miguel and Jerome from school are in the room with me and the lights from the hospital parking lot are making golden stripes on the sheets. The boys are all wrapped up in each other. Their brown beefy shoulders shake and tears fall onto their billboard-size chests. They take me in, the tubes and the wires and the hissing ventilator that breathes for me. Slowly, they kneel at the edge of the bed and place their warm palms in mine, they are so, so warm. I slow blink at them and they cry more because they are witnessing a miracle that I'm too stoned on medicine to understand: I am waking up.

I have spent the past forty-eight hours buckled to a bed in the ICU at Baton Rouge General. All I have in my head are fuzzy flashes of doctors, caged-in fluorescent light bulbs, and the smell of my mom's breath. I know I was in an accident but I don't know how it happened; all I remember is cussing at the CD player in the parking lot of the gas station and wondering if Brian was going to kiss me later. I have a broken neck—the top two vertebrae just under my brain stem, C1 and C2. I have a punctured lung and three busted ribs. My spleen is gone but I never really knew what it was there for, so I don't miss it much. A long, itchy line of staples stretches from my sternum to my pubic bone, and for the past two days, I have been peeing into a bag. Brian is okay, the paramedic is okay, and they think I might be okay, too, but I'll be here for a while because I need a spinal fusion.

My mom comes into the room later that night with Laura. They're carrying Walmart bags and when I attempt to smile at them despite the tube down my throat, their faces crumple into the most beautiful ugliness I've ever seen. Laura's little hummingbird body bounces up and down and she grabs onto my mom's arm. My mom has been sleeping at the hospital with me. They don't have any cots, so she's been living in the waiting room with other sad strangers. Webs of redness cover the whites of her eyes and the supple skin of her cheeks has gone chalk-dry from too much AC. She's undone. She hasn't been undone like this since the day she gave birth to me in a room just like this one.

"Baby, RuRu, Mommy's here."

I attempt another smile for her when she comes closer and she nearly collapses from the joy of it. She has been waiting for me, brushing my hair, singing me songs, and wishing she could travel with me into the jungly space between life and death. Over and over, she traces my face from the bottom of my chin to my forehead and then ski-jumps off the tip of my nose. I bat my gummy lids at her and she belly-laughs. It's like she's just become a mother all over again.

I want to speak to her but I can't, I can't make any sounds with the tube down my throat. I move my fingers a little, just below the restraint, and the motion startles both of us. I uncurl my pointer finger and write *I love you* on the bed with the tip in an invisible ink only she can read. My mom loves Jesus but she was angry at God for a long time, after cancer took her mama when she was just thirteen years old. As she kisses my hands and watches me drift back into sleep, she feels completely loved by him.

When something happens in St. Francisville, people show up. The accident doesn't just happen to me and to my family—it happens to everyone. The entire parish, all colors and classes, all the different people, waits to see me two at a time, loosely corralled by side tables and rows of plastic chairs. They drain the vending machines of Mountain Dew, pass out tins of oatmeal cookies, and fall asleep upright, heads leaning into each other when the caffeine wears off. People who have never spoken before become friends, they share newspapers and snacks, they take care of each other while they take care of me. The West Feliciana High mathematics department comes to visit, Lile's ex-girlfriends, the Ladies in Pearls, Jamise and the Pams, the people from the Episcopal church, the Catholic church, and Frannie's all-day-long church in Hardwood, they all come, even Chuncky, the toughest girl in school, who loves to pick on me and is so imposing that she's never, ever corrected for spelling her own nickname wrong. She makes sure to tell my mom that she's my very best friend, but apparently everyone says that. Still-hot suppers are delivered to my mom nightly in Tupperware steamed all the way up the sides and she tells me there have never been more competing casseroles in one place.

"You are so loved," she says to me, and I hope she knows that she's loved too. She has never been very good at receiving that truth.

My daddy is a celebrity here, so I always know when he arrives; it is the best part of my day. Former students and neighbors mob him when he steps off the elevator, inundating him with hopeful stories, giving him a meal for the Deepfreeze, asking him if there's anything, anything at all they can do to help. He's the man who taught most of them how to show up, the man who at some point showed up for them, for their families. He winds his way out of conversation as politely as he can and turns up the long hallway to my room. He is finally alone with the anticipation of seeing me. His slippery-soled work shoes click and clack on the tile, quicker and louder the closer he gets. Once he crosses the threshold, it's a homecoming for both of us. He holds my hand in his and says, "Pat, pat. Rub, rub. God loves you, Daddy loves you," over and over again and I almost forget that I'm not five years old and beside him in his big bed. I feel peaceful here, held, enveloped by God's love and minded by his angels. My daddy comes often but he can never stay long; sitting next to me as I sit next to death, quiet and still, is too much for him. He leaves so I don't have to see him upset.

Hospital time moves at its own erratic-stopwatch pace, *tick-tick-ticks* between episodes and crises and appointments and surgeries and shifts and dosages. The protocols and routines stretch time in the strangest way and I begin to forget about things outside the hospital, the school assignments I was supposed to turn in, brushing my teeth. They take me off life support; I retch and gag as the thick tube crawls out of places I didn't know I had. My lung collapses again and they put my chest tube back in. It goes straight into my side and I feel every single fiber as it moves through me.

They poke my stomach with needles full of blood thinners that leave pinkish-brown bruises behind; they wait and they monitor. They empty the pee bag, I fill it again. I watch it all lazily, one foot outside my own body on a slow, sleepy opiate trip from a forest of gifted flowers: fluffy carnations and orange lilies shaped like stars, an orchid that I will let die. Even with my mom beside me, the hospital can be a lonely place and sometimes at night when the halls are quiet, I worry that life will never go back to normal.

The cheerleaders come to see me; a blue-and-white oasis of tracksuits and too much blush glows against the ashy walls of the hospital. I can't see them, the doctors are busy fiddling with my chest tube, but they find my mom in the waiting room and surround her with their blueness. They're on the way to a football game in another town but they have stopped by to see me. I should be on the bus with them, cheeks covered in glitter, big bow on the top of my head. They tell my mom with the mad conviction all cheerleaders are made of that they *know* I can get better. Their heads nod, their ponytails flick up and down, their little hands clap reflexively. She visits with them for a bit and they brighten up the sterile tan waiting room with their colorful uniforms.

"Miss Marsha, make sure you watch the nine o'clock news," one of them says on the way out the door.

My mom smiles and squeezes her hand. I should be with them, but instead, I am in a bed with a half-shaved head and atrophied legs.

"And Ruthie Lindsey, a young local girl . . ."

An hour later, I wake up to the sound of my name. My mom is sitting by my shoulder, smiling at the little television in the corner.

Our big-haired local news lady is broadcasting live on the scene from the end zone. The one-man technical team struggles against the noise and the lights and the fury of Friday night football and keeps losing the poor news broadcaster in the crowd. She is wearing a bright blue ribbon in the corner of her blazer, right above her heart. She points to it with a seventeen-tooth grin and explains that it is for me. Then she tells a story I feel like I'm hearing for the first time.

"She had a five percent chance of survival and a one percent chance of walking. . . ."

I take an inventory of my broken bones and missing pieces as she lists them.

The camera slowly pans around the stands and I notice everybody is wearing a blue ribbon; people from my school and this school and other schools, people I know well and people I will never meet. They're saying my name, "Ru-thie, Ru-thie, Ru-thie."

On the opposite edge of the field, I see the cheerleaders. They are clinging to the edges of a big bust-through that says ONLY THE STRONG SURVIVE. THIS ONE'S FOR YOU, RUTHIE. The camera zooms in as a stampede of testosterone rips through it and heads straight for the little news lady, engulfing her. Jerome waves from the field and blows me a kiss. I catch it even though he can't see me. I laugh out loud for the first time and it wakes me, the happy music bounces off the ceiling and for a moment, I'm just a teenager. A Stouffer's Lean Cuisine commercial steals the moment away from me and as the TV lasagna releases big puffs of steam, I know that I need to get back there, to those people.

I've been in the hospital eight days when I'm healthy enough for my spinal fusion. It's almost Thanksgiving now, and though I've been too nauseous from the medicine to eat anything but hunks of bread, I'm suddenly starving. A gob of drool slides out the side of my mouth when I look at the gingerbread cake on the cover of my mom's *Southern Living* and my chest flutters with thoughts of fresh eggs, vegetables from my daddy's garden, the heat of a 400-degree oven, and home. My daddy smiles at me like he's reading my mind. A nurse appears mysteriously at my bedside and wipes the saliva off my chin; the anesthesiologist and the doctor follow.

They talk to my parents while I think about slick, leathery Honey Baked Hams and cookie batter. They draw on my hip in ballpoint pen where they're going to borrow some bone to stabilize the repair in my neck and describe the little wire they're going to use to keep it all together. I'll let them do anything as long as I get to go home. I can hardly hear them talking over the phantom smells of my kitchen.

"Ruthie Lindsey. November 10, 9:42 a.m."

The nurse announces the date and time. My mother's lips graze mine and I start to wilt into the pillow. She's nervous but my daddy stays calm. He sits in his favorite waiting room chair while they operate.

A nurse sits down next to him a few hours later. The procedure is finally over.

"I don't know who you are but your daughter must be somebody special, somebody must really want her here. Her neck popped back into position perfectly when they lifted her onto the table. I've never seen anything like it. We thought we'd need to screw her into a halo brace, but she'll be fine with a traditional one that she can take off in the shower. The bone fusion went wonderfully. Mr. Lindsey, your daughter will be going home soon."

He just smiles, like he knew this would happen all along.

I wake up woozy but entirely myself. My mom cries, crazy from sleep deprivation and relief. My daddy sits next to the bed and holds my hand.

"God loves you, Daddy loves you."

Weeks later, I walk through the sliding doors of the hospital, up a giant neck brace and lots of wire in my neck, down a spleen, and back into my life again.

Sometimes when something bad happens, it's easier to pretend that it didn't.

My daddy cooks his famous barbecue chicken the night I come home.

"Is it the best chicken ever? The best you've ever had?" he asks us, just the way he always does.

My mom makes Sister Schubert's yeast rolls and a bowl of chocolate-chip cookie dough that we eat raw, sticking our spoons right into the sweet muck of it and looking for spiny clusters of pecan. Nobody misses a beat. We curl little ribbon tails for our Christmas presents and listen to Bing Crosby and laugh; we stick to the script that we know. We have lots to say about the accident but no energy or desire to say it. We bury the brokenness and the trauma under an eight-foot spruce tree in the corner. We try to forget—I try hardest of all. We don't get to choose the things that haunt us, the memories that linger, the uninvited feelings that follow us around. We may not want to see them, but eventually they make us look.

I am sitting on the wobbly cream-colored toilet upstairs underneath a Glade PlugIn that smells like cinnamon chewing gum.

I've been home just two days. My mom is making baked beans in the kitchen and Oprah is preaching truth on the living room TV. My daddy is sunk into his chair reading a book as thick as birthday cake about the Cold War. I run the faucet to make sure nobody will hear me and look down at my bruised belly, throbbing away like the diaphragm of a speaker, *bounce, bounce, bounce.* I haven't crapped in twenty-three days. The painkillers slowed everything down and my body kept a tight grip on every ounce of nutrition it could gather in the hospital. Every little stitch and suture on my body is being undone from the pain and the pressure. I hug my knees and a little drop of sweat smacks onto the poodle hair of the bath mat. Everything starts to tremble.

Keep it together. Calm down. You're fine.

I think-pray, *God, Jesus, please!*

I stick my fingernails into my skinny white birch-log legs and leave little half-moon divots behind.

The muscles in my legs seize up, a burning pitches through my pelvis, and I feel myself screaming, just like I did when the bright lights came at me on the road. My panties rip between my knees and I black out. My mom busts through the door and catches me just before my head hits the edge of the tub.

When I come back into the room, she is holding me.

"We have to go back to the hospital, baby," she whispers.

The word *hospital* awakens something in me and I'm part animal. I thrash on the floor and kick against the vanity until the scabs left over from the staples in my stomach begin to weep. I beg her not to take me back.

"Please, Mom! No!"

"Ru, we need to go."

She loads me into the car while I scream and she drives too fast to the ER in Zachary. I catch myself in the rearview mirror, a crazy-eyed skeleton girl.

The nurses give me Xanax and an enema and I tell them all about the time I got diarrhea after going down the waterslide at Blue Bayou. I laugh when the doctor sticks his thumb into my butt and my mom smiles at me through her tears. Just a few hours ago, she was driving me along the same road that almost killed me, trying not to relive every moment of the past month while I made sad coyote sounds in the back seat.

I go home the next morning with stool softeners and nobody says a word about what happened the night before. I shuffle around the house in my neck brace with my butt on fire. We don't talk about the way my mother felt brokenhearted seeing me that way the day before, or the bruises on my arms that are just starting to reveal themselves from where the nurses restrained me. We don't talk about the skeleton girl I saw in the car mirror. It is hard to look back, and we don't want to. Instead, we put *Home Alone* in the VCR and string lights on the tree and let the holidays pass by us, let springtime pass by us. By the end of April, I get my brace off and it's like the accident never happened at all. I graduate on time and get into college.

When they found me slumped over the steering wheel the night of the wreck, there wasn't even a scratch on my skin. I looked pretty and calm, I didn't look like I needed saving but I felt it. I still do.

5

Itty-Bitty Fish

I do college exactly as I'm supposed to. I go to LSU, where every-one in my family goes, and I live with my old friend Susan from the little Christian school in Mississippi. Our room looks like the Ralph Lauren Home display at Dillard's, like J.Crew exploded on a bedspread, and we have a mini refrigerator filled with Diet Dr Peppers and SlimFast. The scented candle we light when we study makes the whole floor smell like lily of the valley. We join the so-rorities that Southern girls are supposed to join and throw parties with fraternities attended by the Southern boys we are supposed to marry. We are a beautiful school of prom queens and cheer-leading captains all swimming the same current our parents and older siblings did, toward marriage at twenty and graduate school at twenty-two and three children by thirty. Everyone loves it here but I'm not sure. I feel like an itty-bitty fish swimming in the wrong direction. Belonging here is drinking too much and having sex and getting bikini waxes. Belonging here is crash dieting, size twenty-six pants, and Cancún on spring break. Belonging here is impossible for me. The other kids party, they get drunk and joyfully lose control. I starve myself because food is the only thing I can control. I play along when I can, I smile big and put gloss on my lips, but I feel an emptiness. There is nothing here that can fill me up but the sugar-free frozen yogurt we all eat to stay skinny.

After the strangeness of freshman year, I'm yearning for the safety of somewhere else, somewhere I know, so I go to work at Camp DeSoto. DeSoto is an overnight summer refuge for second-through tenth-grade girls who love Jesus. It sits high up on top of Lookout Mountain in Mentone, Alabama, where there are so many Christian summer camps, it's hard to hear the crickets over all the acoustic guitars "Kumbaya"-ing through the valley. This is where I spent my summers as a kid, collecting fuzzy friendship bracelets and singing Chickasaw powwow songs I'll never forget that were probably made up by churchy white teenagers in the '80s. Jesus-loving is something that lots of people do in the South, so I do it too. My parents do it and my brothers do it and I'm not sure I know anybody who doesn't do it, who doesn't have a Bible at their bedside or a church they go to on Sunday or a camp just like DeSoto. I apply to be a counselor as soon as I turn eighteen and I convince Katie, my friend from school, to come with me.

Convincing Katie is easy. She lives with me in Miller dorm, the big cream-colored building where all the "best" girls live. It's been slathered with so many coats of neutral paint over the years that the walls are gummy to the touch and pull away in pieces like orange peel. Katie is my best friend, she loves Jesus, and she also needs a summer job. When school lets out, we drive up to Mentone together with the windows rolled all the way down. She talks to me about God as we leave Louisiana and head into Mississippi, where the flat, swampy lowlands start to gain shape. As we enter Appalachia we climb up, up, up, the clouds get low and milky, and the green-leafed forest becomes brittle red pine. When we arrive, we park in the dirt and the dust hits my teeth. I'm met by everything I remember: the sound of branches busting under car tires; the smell of wet bathing suits, evergreen, and Banana Boat; the feeling of home.

"God is good." Katie shuts her eyes and drinks in the scents of pine and lake water through her nose. She looks like she's praying and I begin to wonder if being a Christian is more than just a thing that people do on the weekends.

"God is good," I say back to her, but I'm really just glad to be far away from keg parties and lecture halls and blocking out the sounds of dorm-room sex through saltine-thin walls.

I am entrusted with a cabin of eight preteen girls at DeSoto. They are the perfect mixture of devout and devious and they adore me. There's Sissy, who has two front teeth the size of Starburst candies; Jackie, who hardly speaks at first; and Constance, whose parents are rich with Texas oil money. They're good in the same way that I was, looking to be loved and approved of but also for little flashes of fun. I do my best to let them find their way to harmless mischief, and in exchange, they make me their favorite. They listen to me and respect me and none of the other staff can figure out how I get through to them. My accomplice is a counselor named Leslie, who is as devout and devious as the girls are. Instead of teaching the aerobics class we were assigned, we play Tupac's "California Love" over and over again and let the campers take turns goofy dancing in the center of a big circle. The director can't figure out why everybody is singing songs about the city of Compton but no one gives us away. At night, after lights-out, I go around to each of them and we talk. I ask them how their day was, I tell them they are loved and that they belong. I remember how good it felt to know that when I was younger, how good it still feels now. Then I crawl into bed and let their giggle-whispers go on later than I'm supposed to. I know they are sharing the first secrets of their lives and about an hour after bedtime is the best time to do that. They fall asleep with the blankets kicked off, letting the cool moon shine on their pink skin. Sometimes I hear them praying little prayers and I wonder some more about God and Jesus and how I've ended up here watching their scrawny chests rise and fall. I don't know if I've ever really believed the way they do, the way that Katie does, but I want to, I know I'm supposed to. I say my own little prayer:

Make me be good, make me love Jesus, make me believe.

Morning Watch happens every day down by the lake. We sit in a homemade, cobbled-together amphitheater we call the "worship rocks." It overlooks a big cross sitting on an island in the middle of the lake. At Morning Watch, the counselors take turns sharing chunks of the Bible that they like or telling stories about feeling God's love. Normally I don't listen much, I just wiggle and wait like the campers do, but today is different. A girl my age is standing in front of us—her name is Michelle. She's tall, like me, but her bones are lined with long, graceful muscles and tan outdoorsy skin. She opens her pretty mouth, the sun bounces off the water and covers her in golden dapples, something pulls me toward her, and I can't look away. She tells a story that makes me itch in my skin about hating herself and learning to love herself again through Jesus. It's painful and embarrassing, but she isn't ashamed. She knows that she belongs and she knows that she's loved. I look around at the other girls: tears are falling freely, sliding down burnt-butter cheek skin and smacking onto the dirt. They all carry a part of her sadness for her and nurture the words from her. It feels safe and tender, like home. I let tears warm my own cheeks. This is where I belong.

I say my prayer again: *Make me be good, make me love Jesus, make me believe.*

It's just past 7 a.m. on Wednesday when I bust into Katie's messy cabin. In two days, I'm supposed to lead Morning Watch and talk to the whole camp about why I believe and how much I love Jesus but I haven't even found him yet. Since that day on the worship rocks, I've been searching for him everywhere—I look into the polished silver of the lake and think about it on the walk through the thick part of the forest that smells like fire and hot dogs. All I can see in the lake is my too-lumpy body and all I can think about on my walks is burning calories.

Katie is sitting in a nest of camp linens journaling furiously and twirling her mud-colored ponytail. She doesn't look at all surprised to see me when the door swings open.

"I don't have a Jesus story. I'm talking on Friday but I don't have a Jesus story."

I fall onto the empty mattress across from hers and bury my head into the citronella-soaked pillow. I cough and she waves me over to join her in the blanket nest.

"Ruthie," she says, baffled, "you have a Jesus story. You *are* a Jesus story."

Her eyes are looking into mine as far as they can, searching for some recognition. There's none.

"Your accident. God chose to save you."

The accident.

It has only been a year and a half but I hardly think about it. Katie grabs my hand and looks at me with absolute certainty.

"You're alive, Ruthie. You are proof of the Lord's love."

It all makes so much sense. I've never asked for the reason why it happened but now I have one. At 7:22 a.m. in Katie's musty green cabin, I rebaptize myself with two sprays of her Clinique Happy perfume and I get a warm, holy, grapefruit-scented feeling all over me.

On Friday morning, I stand with the big cross in the background and talk about what happened to me. I know the words are romantic and I like the way it sounds when me, God, and Jesus are the main characters in my story, three divine musketeers. The sun warms my back like my daddy's hand while I speak and the girls are patient, like they were with Michelle. They listen graciously and don't rush me through when I talk about how scared I was and how grateful I am to be alive. I'm fully exposed, imperfections and fears strung up and flapping in the wind, but instead of shame, I feel so much love. I don't know it yet, but this moment will serve as my anchor in so many ways. Later, when I'm lost, unsure, or alone, I will learn to look up and around for those journeying with me. I will learn to let them carry me when I'm weak and I will learn to hold their weight when I'm strong. The power of community will shape, astound, and sustain me.

After I finish my story, Leslie and Katie rest their hands in mine and I lead a clumsy prayer; we bow our heads all together as the tall trees moan like cattle in the breeze behind us. I haven't found Jesus, but I've found fellowship and I believe in it with all my heart. I devote myself to it. I'm not unhappy when I return to LSU, but after fall semester, I transfer to Ole Miss, where Leslie goes to school. I feel called there, like all the answers to my questions about God exist in leafy Oxford, Mississippi. I sink myself deep into college ministry.

Ole Miss is everything I want it to be, a giant golf course–green space filled with friends to collect, all sprawled out on big blankets watching the sky. It's warm and wonderful and people love me. It's high school all over again but with no parents and slightly bigger boobs. I join the Reformed University Fellowship with Leslie: RUF is the cool Christian group on campus. We talk about philosophy and listen to good music and don't flutter around campus with rubbery WWJD bracelets the way the nerdy "Christian crusaders" do. We sing worship songs, but we sing dirty rap too. Most nineteen-year-olds would feel stifled by conservative Presbyterianism, but I feel liberated, like I've finally found my people. Jesus is still missing in action but I claim him as my savior. I yearn for him and search frantically for a sign of him in potholes and bags of potato chips and cloud shapes. After two years of Bible study and RUF, I'm still waiting for my own testimony. I try to be the best Christian I can, to invite Jesus into my life, but I'm not the best Christian. Laura Treppendahl is.

There is a story about Laura Treppendahl that people in Baton Rouge like to tell. In high school speech class, she has to give a presentation on something she's passionate about and she chooses the dangers of drunk driving. She stands at the podium under a laminated poster of the American flag and delivers her argument beautifully, eloquently, even. Her big, shiny gem eyes glow with truth and she gets a mighty applause afterward that lasts two whole minutes. She begins the walk back to her seat when the teacher announces that for the next assignment, the class will have to present the opposing case to whatever they gave their speech on. The room goes silent.

The very idea of advocating *for* such a sad and sinful thing breaks poor Laura's heart and she's horrified to tell her mother, Coco, after school. Coco listens to her daughter's worries and smiles, promising her that everything will be fine.

"You'll figure it out." She smiles. That's exactly what Laura does.

The following week, she stands at the podium in speech class once again and tells the story of a wonderful young girl who loved Jesus and everyone and everything with all her heart. Tragically, shockingly, she was killed by a drunk driver leaving a bar in his truck on a Tuesday evening. At the girl's funeral, Laura says, the gospel was proclaimed and many people came to know and love Jesus, many people were saved. Even in tragedy if you open your heart to the Lord, there can be triumph. Again, she speaks beautifully and eloquently, and again, she gets a hefty applause from the class.

Years later, I will hear the story from Miss Coco herself and I'll feel the aching love she has for her daughter as she tells it to me. I can't see past the sadness of it all. I can't see beyond the girl in her casket who shouldn't be there. I can't see what Laura Treppendahl sees, but I want to.

Laura is a freshman. She arrives at the beginning of my senior year. She walks right up to me after attending her first RUF meeting and knocks me out with her light.

"You're Ruthie," she announces before she even thinks to introduce herself.

Katie told me I would fall in love with her and she was right. Years of joy have built a dimple into her right cheek and given her doe eyes little crinkles in the corners. She's beautiful—gorgeous, actually—but it's as though she's never noticed it herself, never even thought to check. She holds my hand gently in hers when she speaks, and even though she is three years younger than I am, she seems older. I let her pull my hand to her heart and she holds it there to rest on top of the gentle patter; it's like holding on to a rabbit.

"I heard about your accident," she sings. "You were on our prayer list for almost a year at church but I prayed for you so much longer than that, I was called to, I just knew it. I'm so glad that we're friends now. God is so good."

I look at her glowing at me, cheeks lifting up into two pink circles. She's so loving, so pure. I've never met anybody like her. I've never met anybody I want to be more like.

As the year chugs along, I watch her shine eclipse my own. People say we are two peas in a pod, that Laura is just like me, but they're wrong. She lives out of an abundance of love; I live out of a hunger for it. Her goodness flows over campus like hot honey, and for the first time in my life, I'm envious of someone. I watch her sing "Holy, Holy, Holy," chin tilted toward God, cheeks glowing with joy. I watch her give and give and give with utter selflessness. I try to learn from her, make my own competing version of her specialness, but I can't. She's sustained by the love of Jesus. Whatever that love is, whatever it feels like, I can't imagine it would ever be enough for me.

When I finish senior year, I get a job in Nashville, Tennessee. I'm going to be an assistant youth group leader at a Presbyterian church near where Leslie's parents grew up. Laura is ecstatic when I tell her about it. She grabs my hands and holds them at her heart again and says she'll be praying for me. I know that she will be. I drive up to Tennessee all by myself and think about her on the way. I wonder if someone who doesn't see Jesus can teach him and I wonder if wanting to know his love is enough to speak of it. When a little girl with a dimple on her cheek waves at me through her car window on the interstate, I see Laura in her and decide it's a sign. I keep driving and I keep searching.

One year later, Laura Treppendahl will be killed by a drunk driver. She will only be nineteen years old. Her body won't look broken on the outside, but her insides will slide into each other. She will die instantly. Her injuries will be far less punishing than mine were on paper, but for some reason, I will be the one to watch them bury her little body not far from the cemetery where they would have buried mine. I will stop trying to find Jesus when I hear the news, but when I go to her visitation in Baton Rouge and see the lines filling the streets and trickling into the sanctuary of the church, I'll remember the mysterious, breathtaking love that envelops us. I'll remember the sunlight that poured from her eyes when she prayed. I'll remember the story she told in speech class. The day of her funeral, the gospel will be proclaimed and so many people will come to know the love God has for them.

I'll keep searching and searching for truth, for God, and for little bits of Laura in the world.

6

Sex, Drums, and Dido

Jack wears snap-front cowboy shirts and blue jeans that bell out over the top of his New Balance tennis shoes. He has just enough patches of beard across his cheeks and chin to make him look grown-up, but I can tell when he smiles that there are parts of him that are still very young and will probably stay that way forever. I have those parts too. His eyes are two bowls of hot brownie batter and he is gloriously, perfectly, miraculously taller than I am. I know almost right away that I could love him.

When we first meet, I'm living in a very beige upstairs apartment off Belmont Boulevard in Nashville. It's within throwing distance of a sushi restaurant that serves bright green martinis and a university music school. The area is populated almost exclusively by its students, someday songwriters and budding rock stars whose parents insisted they get an education. I live with a girl named Caroline whom I met freshman year at LSU. She works as a lobbyist; outside of wearing lots of pantsuits and talking about "the Capitol," I have no idea what a lobbyist actually does. Living with Caroline automatically gifts me a million new built-in friendships, and even though Katie and Leslie have both ended up in Nashville, too, the whole point of living in a big city is to meet as many people as possible, so I lap it up. Caroline also comes with a musician boyfriend named Griffin, who lives with us when they're getting along. He writes songs like an old man from coal country but he's from Ohio and he's only twenty-three.

It's a Friday afternoon in September. I'm sitting on our doughy couch, which is just a few shades of beige darker than the walls, and three-year-old Kate Dortch is painting my nails with a green apple–scented marker. I make almost as much money babysitting on Friday nights as I do assisting the youth minister on Sunday mornings, so I keep my weekends booked solid with toddler manicures and dress-up games. Little Kate is my favorite. She's allowed to get dirty and wear whatever she wants to because her mom is open-minded and loves for her to play. Today, she has chosen two different shoes, pajama bottoms, and a backward pirate costume. Griffin and Caroline love her too; they pop their heads out of the bedroom, where they have been having a serious discussion about their relationship, to admire the latest questionable outfit choice. We all agree that she has outdone herself and she lights up like a Christmas star.

"My Roosie," she says, exasperated, shoving a yellow marker at me and sticking out her hand. Her fingernails are the size of the buttons on our television remote. I pop off the lid, draw a heart on her palm that she oooooohs over. I imagine my own future kids in moments like these and I know that I'll be a good mom someday.

Just as I'm about to begin on her nails, the door rattles in its frame and somebody knocks on it. I can tell it's a man from the deep sound his throat makes when he nervously clears it; I can tell he's a young man by the fact that he needs to clear it at all. Kate looks at me, hand stretched out, begging me not to get up, but the knock comes again so I leave her devastated in the tan cushions.

He says his name is Jack, and in those first wonderful seconds, I have never heard a more perfect word or seen a more perfect person. He's Griffin's drummer, and as I hear his thunder-boom voice I sink another inch deeper into loving him. I just stare for a second and don't say anything. It's all I can manage to do.

"Roosie!" Kate calls impatiently from the couch.

She is standing up with her hands on her hips, forgotten and deeply offended. Jack smiles at her and she stares at her feet.

"I'm Ruthie, I live here."

It's a bad introduction, but it just pops out.

I force my hand into his and it gets hot right away. The feeling of him travels down my legs and buzzes in the arches of my feet.

Griffin emerges from the bedroom and embraces Jack with one of those hollow thumps to his back that boys give to each other and they tuck themselves into the kitchen nook to discuss something urgent about music. I hand Kate three uncapped markers to play with so that I can watch Jack's dark eyebrows rise and fall as he talks. She squeals, an oblivious bundle of pink smiley fat rolls coloring all over herself, relieved to have her "Roosie" back from the strange man. Jack's eyes drift over to mine every few seconds. I can feel them on me and I wish Kate was fifteen years older so that we could quietly gossip about what was happening.

He stuffs a CD of Griffin's newest music into his backpack and they say goodbye with another thump. When he rounds the corner of the nook, our eyes lock. Neither of us knows what we're supposed to do next.

"It was nice to meet you, Ruthie."

"Nice to meet you, Jack."

He leaves but I know I'll see him again. My heart is sure.

Only about fifty-two hours pass until I find myself by his side. The bowling alley is a still, heavy cloud of flat beer and Odor-Eaters, but to me, it could be Paris. Jack is here. He and Griffin are leaving in the morning for a monthlong tour and all their friends have gathered to send them off with plastic jugs of Bud Light and rented shoes. Griffin and Caroline were supposed to come with me but they decided to stay home to argue, make up, and argue again.

Jack stands up from his plastic seat when he sees me and begins walking toward me as I walk toward him. I weave between groups of kids eating cheese fries, he dodges the line for the bathroom; I slip a little where the carpet turns to tile, he ducks under a low-hanging SNACK BAR sign. Finally, we meet under a giant television screen illuminated with other people's bowling scores. He puts his arms around me the way we both wanted him to at the apartment and his chest feels exactly the way I've been hoping it would, like such a safe place. The crowd thins for us a bit as he leads me to his lane with a hand against the small of my back. I have seen boyfriends do this to girlfriends before and I can hardly believe it is happening to me.

The noise of the night is constant, giant marbles rolling and smashing and being swallowed into black shadow. We tell our stories, a formality of falling in love with someone, shifting in our uncomfortable plastic bucket seats and wishing they weren't bolted to the floor. He's from Houston, he has two brothers, and he's a little bit younger than I am. His mom's name is Sandra and she worries too much, she wants him to meet a nice girl (I decide, without hesitation, that this is directed at me). He laughs when I tell him about living on a farm, about driving the old truck down the road at twelve years old, and about my daddy plowing the garden with Amos the mule. It's work to make our legs touch but we do it because we *have* to, because there is simply too much space between us. I can see my pulse throbbing through my jeans at the knee and the sight of our thighs next to each other is so overwhelming and exciting I almost need to get up and leave. We miss our turns, every turn, and the others give up on us. At the end of the night, Jack walks me to my car across the big empty dark of the parking lot and I lay my cheek on his shoulder. We say goodbye.

"Good to see you, Ruthie."

"Good to see you, Jack."

I don't sleep at all when I get home. I think about what it will be like to kiss him and wonder how in the world I'll be able to wait an entire month to do it. I do wait, though, sitting out on the roof and mapping out our future. When he does get back, he doesn't call. I'm surprised and I'm sad but I keep waiting. My heart is so sure of him.

It's just before Thanksgiving and Jack is onstage. He is surrounded by an actual halo of flash-bright stage lights, fiddling with his drum kit. We're at a club called 3rd and Lindsley. It's in an industrial area of town, stuck right in the glow of the freeway lights and a giant fluorescent strip club sign. It's one of the best places in the city for a young band to play, and in just a few minutes, Griffin will be on. Leslie is with me, I made her come, and together, we stare at Jack from behind a basket of fried pickles and wonder if he's noticed me.

The guitars make a loud sound and the lights go down. Griffin walks up to the mic and begins to sing a gorgeous song about the rain that everybody loves, even Leslie, but I can hardly hear any of it; the only music I can hear is the music that Jack's making. He thuds and throbs, makes a series of wonderful clattering crashes from his little leather stool behind the drum kit. I can feel the joy pouring out of him and onto me. He closes his eyes and concentrates, letting his arms travel all over. I close my eyes too and take it in. I know as I listen to him and sway along that we'll be together.

After the set is over, I find him standing alone by the bar, staring into the foamy bottom of a pint glass. His mahogany eyes are sunk deep into his skull. He is skinnier than I remember him; there's a heaviness all around him that I hadn't noticed before. He doesn't look like he wants to talk to anyone and my heart is so sure that I don't mind waiting another month or twelve for him to be ready. I go to leave, but as I push through the crowd his eyes find me again and a glimmer of him returns. I walk straight into his chest and I think he knows that we'll be together too.

We go to an after-party together where we talk about the holidays, my mom's dressing, and his mom's pie. He laughs and it is the best music either of us hears the whole night: whatever was broken in him suddenly isn't anymore. His uncooperative, horsetail-thick hair falls into his eyes and he holds my hand. When everybody leaves at 3 a.m., we go to a Waffle House, where we first sit in the parking lot and listen to a Dido record he thinks is romantic. I make him try my smothered hash browns, which he says look like cat barf, and he feeds me a bite of pancake. The sun begins to come up and we both nearly miss our flights home to see our families. When he comes back from his trip, he becomes the first boyfriend I, at twenty-three years old, have ever had.

We fall in love like a pair of diving seabirds, nose-down, at top speed, totally fearless, and we parade our newfound love around town with kisses on the street and double dates. I watch him play drums from the side of the stage and I'm so proud to be with him I could bust open. I love him the way I like to be loved; I delight in him. Jack has never been delighted in this way by a girl he likes and he thinks it's the best feeling in the world. I go to Houston to meet his parents and he meets mine. Then they meet each other and we start to dive harder and faster. The heaviness he had that night at the club still comes back to him some days, but I never let him sit in it alone. We binge-watch *24* and sleep late and order cheese sticks from Domino's while Kiefer Sutherland walks slowly around corners with his gun pointed. I don't know why Jack gets sad, but I like that I make him feel better. I'm special and needed, I belong.

We've been dating four months when he tells me that the thing that makes him sad is depression. We're at my apartment and the weather is bad; the sky is brown and the Channel Five news team tells us to get in our safe spot. I'm already in mine. My cheek is at its home on Jack's shoulder and he starts in when the weather girl is done showing off the splotchy radar shape. He tells me he doesn't really know why it happens, that maybe it's trying to make everybody happy, or being a talented musician in a town of tens of thousands of talented musicians. Maybe it's having an unspeakably successful father, or having ADHD. It could just be the weather. Thunder crunches right after he says this and we both giggle. He waits for me to react, to ask worried questions or ask to see the medicine he takes, but I don't. He could have the bubonic plague and I'd still love him till the day I died.

65

"It's okay," I tell him. "You're not alone. You don't ever have to be."

I don't know why I say it, but it seems to be exactly what he needs to hear. His cheek finds its way onto my shoulder now, and I comb through his hair with my fingers, rubbing little circles on his temples. The storm stops, the sun begins to peek at us through the green-studded branches of the trees outside the window, and we become something more than just kids kissing on the sidewalk. We dive even faster, even deeper, into loving each other.

Love feels nothing like they told me it would. It's nothing like the calm, comfortable kiss my daddy puts on my mom's forehead; it's nothing like the humble, kind, patient union they talked about in RUF. Love is rocket fuel and I can never get enough of it. I've only ever kissed a few boys before Jack, but everything is different with him. I want him. I can hardly keep my clothes on when he parks his clunky tan Expedition by the curb, and though we're both saving ourselves until marriage, we do everything, see everything, and touch everything until we have traveled every inch inside the boundaries the church set for us. We roll around for hours under my big white duvet, lanky bodies knotted together, hot, heavy animal breathing making the sheets wet. I feel so much happiness and so much shame as I watch him sleeping naked beside me and I wonder if there are other church leaders splayed out in their underwear promising God they won't let their boyfriends go down on them next time. At least not for as long. I'm supposed to be good, it's my job to be good, but I can't stay good anymore.

It starts out like it normally does. We're up late in Jack's barren room, almost as naked as the walls are. I kiss him and he presses himself into me. I take his face in both hands and kiss him again. He unsnaps my bra and his hands move over me. I put my hands on him. Our bodies start to make the motions without us asking them to, and I tell him to keep going. He pulls my panties off and we get lost. We know nothing about sex. Nobody told us about our bodies, how powerful they are, that they can demand things. All they told us in school and church was not to listen to them if they spoke. He puts himself in me for just a second but we stop ourselves, panting, zapped into submission like a pair of bad suburban dogs caught in the invisible fence. The guilt is a shock wave. I run to the bathroom and bleed onto toilet paper; I'm not a virgin. Jack's face is white when I climb back into the bed. I pull my underwear up to my belly button and start to cry. I return to twelve, hiding in the bathroom at the slumber party with covered ears, waiting until the other girls stopped talking about what it would feel like to be touched.

"Tell me everything is going to be okay," I sniff at him.

He kisses the top of my head and his mouth quivers. "Everything is going to be okay. I love you. I love you so much."

He says it because he *does* love me, but also because of what we've done and who we are and where we come from. We know the rules: the person you have sex with is the person whom you marry; the person you say "I love you" to is the person whom you marry. So we both silently agree that's what we should do.

"I love you too," I whisper.

We kiss and feel forgiven. Over the next few weeks, shame chases desire in a giant circle.

We get engaged quickly and none of it, really, is a surprise. I go on a mission trip to Mexico that I almost miss because I'm sick from taking a Plan B. We had been fooling around and even though he finished into a throw pillow, I was worried I might get pregnant. When I get back to Nashville, sunburnt and still nauseous, Jack claims to be stuck working in the studio, so he sends his grinning, winking roommate to pick me up. He drops me off by the curb and honks the horn three very precise times as I lug my suitcase to the front door. When I climb up the stairs to our apartment, there is a note outside:

TAKE YOUR SHOES OFF.

I smile big. I know what I'm about to see. I kick off my sneakers and open the door.

Rose petals, shiny and red as apple skins, are sprinkled all over the shitty gray carpet. They meander through a village of votive candles and lead into my bedroom. Ray Lamontagne is playing from my little stereo speakers at the end of the bed. He's singing about the woman who redeemed him.

I take it in, walking slow, squishing my feet into the petals and making pink streaks that won't ever come out of the carpet, passing mounds of melted wax that won't ever come out either, and moving with the music. Step by step by step, the shame starts to lift from me.

He is there on his knee in the almost-dark, a cluster of faraway candles on the nightstand are lighting his face just enough to let me see his perfect, quivering lips. The room is covered in new dresses from my favorite boutique; I'll get to pick one to wear out for our celebration. I smile at him and I keep walking. He doesn't know anything about dresses and I assume he must have had help. As I get closer, his great-grandmother's diamond makes glimmering stars on the wall and I notice him turning it nervously in his hands. It could be anything, really, a rubber band, a Ring Pop, I don't care, I just want to wear it. He tells me that he loves me again and his eyes fill with tears.

"Ruthie, will you marry me?"

I can hardly speak but I say enough of a yes. We hold each other and my cheek settles in its favorite place against him. We let Ray sing us another song and we rock back and forth, not really dancing, just hanging on while the music carries us for three minutes.

We barely know each other, we barely know ourselves, but we make new promises to erase the ones that we broke. After we make them, we feel a wonderful relief that we don't talk about and pretend isn't there. I call my parents, who have been waiting by the phone, and Jack calls his. I pick out a new dress and we go to a restaurant that serves cheese plates and champagne, and as we spread buttery slabs of Brie onto hunks of bread, faces bathed in candlelight, we build a life together with our words. I dream up the little house we will buy and the dog that will teach us how to be parents; Jack talks about seeing the world together and we commit to only buying real Christmas trees. We play a little game of house.

That night, I fall asleep in Caroline's bed and he sleeps in mine. We're pretending to be virgins again, we're course correcting even though we're engaged. I look up at the ceiling and think about picket fences and Christmas trees and babies and wonder if marrying someone is just playing a game of house that lasts forever. The heaviness that Jack knows finds me. I'm scared and lonely, even though I'll never be alone again. Maybe it's always trying to do the right thing, or growing up. Maybe it's the hormones left over from the Plan B. I don't think it has anything to do with the weather.

7

Southern Baptist Romance

There is a church down the road from my family's farm. Only about two handfuls of people can fit inside, and once a month, they have a Sunday service at 6:30 a.m. that my mom loves. This quiet, humble, gunmetal-gray building tucked up in the trees off Old Laurel Hill Road is where I become Jack's wife. This is where *we* begin.

When I was a little girl, I wanted to invite a thousand people to my wedding; I wanted two thousand eyeballs glued to me all day long and a horse and a carriage and a sheet cake from Baskin-Robbins as big as a dog bed. I wanted to hear a thousand gasps at the same time when I walked into the church and my special song started to play. During Communion, I practiced what it would be like, plucking up the edges of my church dress and walking slowly between the pews toward my cracker and wine. *Right, stop. Left, stop. Right, stop. Left, stop.* The pastor smiled at me and I smiled back. He was my handsome husband in this game, even though he looked a bit like a tree frog. When I got back home, I changed into my shiniest leotard for the big party that came after the procession and I slow danced by myself, arms straight out, resting on a pair of invisible shoulders. The spotted dogs watched me sway and I serenaded them with Madonna's "Crazy for You." It reverberated through the forest and made the birds fly away. To be watched is to be wanted and to be wanted is to be loved. I closed my eyes and daydreamed it, the dress, the dancing, the desire, as hard as I possibly could.

When I actually do get married, there are no horses or ice-cream cakes. There is no Madonna. Only a couple of dozen people are invited to behold me when I walk down the aisle, and the only set of eyeballs I care about belongs to the shivery, nervous man who waits for me at the end of it. Little Ruthie would be bored; she would wrinkle her nose at the smell of the great-granddaddy chapel, the old songbooks, and the soft, rotten wood. She wouldn't understand the quiet sacredness of it all, but she doesn't have a say. Little Ruthie doesn't cross this threshold with me.

The morning of the wedding is like a coffee commercial, misty and thoughtful and just cold enough for a sweater—though in Louisiana, sweater weather never lasts past 9 a.m. My mom kisses my head and drives to the church early to supervise the position-ing of fat white roses and stalks of leather-leaf fern. This is as much her day as it is mine; it's the gift she's been waiting to give me my whole life. The wait has not been easy for her. Lile says that when I was in college and not dating anybody, she convinced herself I was a lesbian and openly mourned the loss of planning a perfectly picturesque, abundantly heterosexual ceremony for me. Today, she finally gets to play her opus. I don't really care about the tiny wedding, the details, the buttercream or ganache, the huge reception, or the plantation with the good picture-taking tree, so I give all of it to her and watch her devour it.

The dress hangs in a bag on a puffy pink hanger. It sits there all morning just staring at me from the back of my parents' bedroom door. It's jawbone white and cost only $250; Katie took me to the Nicole Miller store at the mall and we found it in the bridesmaid's section next to a big stack of marked-down platform shoes. It's perfect, unembellished, stark, and simple. The bottom swings with me when I dance, and the bodice droops all the way down in the back, allowing the space just above my butt to peek out through a tiny window of scalloped lace.

I smile when I take it down and step into it, when it's almost time for us to go to the church. It grasps my torso just enough to make me feel like a woman. I pat powder on my cheeks, draw a perfect line around my lips, and stare at myself in the mirrored cove of the vanity. I'm ready. I know I should savor the motions of this day but I just want to be married, I just want to be with Jack, made whole in him the way God thinks a woman should be. I don't want to feel shame for the body inside the white dress anymore, and after today, our sinfulness, our lust, will become sacredness.

My daddy is too giddy to speak when I walk onto the porch and he sees me in my white not-wedding dress and bare toes. I'm half grown-up, half baby girl, and it makes him squeal. He fans his fingers out like sunbeams, steps back, and just stares at me. He's wanted today for me as long as my mom has; wanted me to be loved the way that Jack loves me, wanted me to have babies, wanted me to know the joy that he knows, the endless unbroken love of family. A part of him is made whole today, too, three children, all married, all sworn to the right partner, to godliness, and to righteousness. My happiness is his total absolution, for the war, for recovering from the war, for hard work in the hot sun, for raising his children right. This is what he has prayed for and he knew it would come. While my mom worried about the declining population of single white men with good jobs, my daddy just shook his head and laughed, and when Jack asked for his blessing, he knew exactly what to say: "If Ruthie chooses you, you must be very special."

We ride to the church together. My daddy drives and I sit beside him in his big, boat-shaped car, which he had cleaned just for this trip up the road. It feels like the beginning of a new school year. He's all shined up and he's chosen my favorite yellow bow tie. I'm excited and wearing too much lipstick. Childhood is a green smear in the window as we go bumping along the gravel through the country where so much of me happened: the lake I swam in, the fields where I braided stalks of Indian grass, the old hunting camp where I used to hide out and watch for deer poking their noses out of the forest. I say goodbye to childhood, in a way, giving it a five-minute funeral as we roll along. My daddy looks with me, fence drifting into fence, the road getting narrower. He's smiling so hard that his little round glasses rest on the top of his cheeks instead of the bridge of his nose. There are wise words he could say, but instead he just pats the top of my hand with his fingertips and peers down at my engagement ring. Neither of us has gotten used to it being there. I wish he would grab my fingers and wiggle them the way he used to when I was eight years old and we were driving to WCCA. I wish he would shimmy and be silly with me just one more time. It could be a last dance together, for just the two of us.

A spit of trees juts out, and on the other side are parked cars. We slow; my daddy looks outside at the green smear and sighs. He says goodbye to my childhood too.

"God loves you, Daddy loves you." He smiles his perfect smile at me.

I walk barefoot into the church through the tall, arched doorway. There is a spray of flowers on the door but very little on the inside. Holy places like these don't need decorations, just enough sun to illuminate the dust flecks left over from the Civil War and enough space to let people see the notches in the wood, to drink in her quiet glory. My special song begins to play and my daddy and I start down the aisle. We walk the way I practiced so many times before as a child. *Right, stop. Left, stop.* The 150-year-old floorboards creak low and quiet under us and everybody's eyes are on me, even those of my daddy, who's as proud as a peacock and wishing our walk could last forever. Our friends from Nashville are singing to us, Ian on the pump organ and Matthew on guitar. They grin at me and I grin back, hoping I don't look like a beekeeper in my veil. My gaze is forward and Jack is waiting for me. He's a bit past the pews in a dusty yellow spotlight the sun makes just for him. I get a happy little stomachache when I see him seeing me; his lips are quivering so hard I don't know if he'll be able to speak. He's clean-shaven, and I realize I've never seen his cheeks before. He has half a dimple I didn't know was there and he looks like a little boy, a sweet child. In so many ways, we are still children. When we reach him, my daddy lets go of my hand and for one bittersweet moment it just hangs there. Then he places it gently into Jack's and looks straight into my eyes.

"God loves you, Daddy loves you." He says it for me just one more time, lifting a corner of organza to kiss me on the forehead and then fading back into the crowd of loved ones. Everything becomes white noise.

Fifteen minutes later, I am Mrs. Ruthie Moore. We kiss and we dance and we go to Mexico. We do everything the way we are supposed to.

When we get back to start life together, marriage is a sweet but clumsy stumble through firsts. God continues to offer us rules but no instructions. He says love is patient, love is kind, but he doesn't tell us how to touch each other or open a joint checking account or piece each other back together after the falling aparts of life. He just tells us to grow old together without teaching us to grow up. We buy a pretty yellow house across from a coffee shop. I fill it with beautiful things: antiques from St. Francisville, flea-market furniture, and puffy throw pillows. We get the little dog and we call her Ellie. Giving her a human name, we think, will better prepare us for having a human baby. But not for a few years. We are young and we are hopeful. We have a home, two bedrooms and a backyard and crown molding, but we don't know how to reach each other once we're living inside it.

We promised God that we would take care of and honor each other but we don't even know how to do those things for ourselves. The game of house we play is less about communication and more about conservation. I want Jack to cut the lawn the way my daddy did. I want him to fix things, to be a leader, to love the church—the things I know men do. He doesn't and I don't say anything. Jack wants me to roast chicken and mash potatoes the way his mom did; he wants me to mother him a little and to do the shopping—the things he knows women do. I don't even know how to work the gas stove and all we have in our cupboards are big bags of M&M's and Gushers that I pick up from the Walgreens. He doesn't say anything to me either. God says love doesn't get angry or hold grudges, so we don't talk about any of it, our secret expectations, the way things were for us growing up and the way we want them to be. We hire a lawn guy named Todd and order takeout instead of being mad. We outsource. Nobody wants to rock a boat that's been pushed out to the middle of the sea.

God says that we are one flesh now but we don't feel that way. I decorate our bedroom with my grandmother's vanity and a grown-up-looking sleigh bed from Pottery Barn but we don't know how to reach each other inside it either. Once the adrenaline of skin against skin begins to dull, the sex we've been waiting for doesn't feel good. Not for either of us. I lie there with frightened-rabbit eyes as Jack rocks on top of me. I try to look sexy, shut my eyes and flip my hair back. I climb on top of him one time, which he thinks is the hottest thing that has ever happened, but we are both so embarrassed when he uses the word *hot* that we can hardly concentrate. We try, we kiss, and we roll around, but we bring our luggage with us to bed, the things we want to talk about but don't, the little drops of anger that we swallow to keep the peace, the weight of a life together.

After years spent listening to the stories the church tells about a woman's body, mine still feels like contraband. I don't know how to feel pleasure without shame, I don't know how to touch myself without feeling like a vandal, I don't know what to tell Jack. I know less about my vagina than he does, and even if I did know what the word *clitoris* meant, I couldn't tell him what to do with it or where to find it. I give him no guidance at all and he doesn't guide me either. We become very polite, very quiet lovers, because love is not self-seeking, love is always on its best behavior.

Even though there is clumsiness and stumbling through this season, there is also dancing and laughter. The moments where we forget the promises we made and the big, adult future we're responsible for building are pure joy. We adore each other, delight in each other, and smile so hard our faces start to look older. We eat tacos at midnight and go to matinee movies at the Belcourt Theatre; we have friends who love us and careers that we're proud of. We sit on the back porch and listen to music for hours. Jack still has heavy days, but I learn how to make him feel better; I slip in beside him under the covers at 3 p.m, drape myself over him like a blanket, and let him sleep all day. He learns how to make me feel better too—he takes me out dancing even when he doesn't want to, and he lets me have all the attention. We love each other the best that we can. We try to do marriage the way we think our parents did it and our pastors did it so that we can become whole like they are. It never occurs to either of us, to anyone, that our parents, our wisest teachers, the ones who wove our moral fabric and covered us up in it, could have done it all wrong.

We find out about Sam three months after we get married. Sam is Jack's father; he's charming and successful and knows exactly how impressive he is. He has the sheen of a fancy game show host, but instead of reading trivia on daytime television, he is a renowned litigator. He wins awards and gives speeches at events and makes so much money that sometimes he sends us checks in the mail for absolutely no reason at all. It's his love language, as far as I can tell. Jack respects, fears, loves, and hates him all at once, and they look the exact same: same height; big, dark brows; and wide, wolfish smiles. Though they're each other's perfect duplicate, standing in the space around them feels so different to me—it always has.

We're looking after the house and children of one of the preachers at my church when Jack's oldest brother calls. The kids are happy-screeching upstairs and we're leaning against a big granite slab in the kitchen, imagining that this place and its happy kid sounds belong to us. We've just begun talking about the future and now we're trying it on, taking our game of house to the next level. I sprinkle cheese powder the color of traffic cones on top of noodles from a box and squelch it around the bottom of a too-big pot while Jack watches and smiles, shocked that I figured out where they keep the cookware and how to use it. His phone vibrates while I'm stirring.

"Hey," Jack says to the phone, and he disappears through the French doors to the patio.

The kids come into the kitchen all bouncy and sugar-filled and I mound their "dinner" onto plates that are probably meant for special occasions. They smile big at me—the oldest just lost a tooth and the youngest is jealous—and they fling questions at the back of my head while bad news quietly unfolds outside.

"Can we have Pop-Tarts?"

"Can we watch *Shrek*?"

"When will I get a mustache?"

I walk to the glass and tap on it but Jack ignores me. He rakes his hand through his hair and big clouds of steam escape from his nose. His lips are zipped into a straight line.

The kids keep bouncing and asking questions.

"Do you want to hear a joke?"

"How many popsicles can we have?"

"Can we put on a show?"

When they've slurped up their little hills of macaroni, I sit them in front of an animated movie about friendly Protestant vegetables and I go back to my window to watch and wonder about Jack.

Twenty minutes later, when an asparagus is learning a Bible story about Sarah and Abraham, he comes back in.

"My dad is leaving."

He says it like a little boy, like they're all still living together in the big white house in Texas and Christmas is going to be ruined this year. His lips are quivering like they were just a few months ago at our wedding, the wedding where Sam hammered on the side of his glass with a fork and gave a speech in front of our friends and family about the sanctity of it all. He talked about his wife, Sandra, whom he called beautiful and kind, and who smiled up at him adoringly as he spoke. I looked at my parents, holding hands and nodding in agreement with every word. I grabbed for Jack's hand and squeezed it: we listened too. Sam raised his flute above his plate of fat Gulf shrimp and kissed Sandra on the mouth. It was one of the last kisses he would give to her.

"They're getting divorced," Jack says. "It's over. I can't believe it."

I don't know what to do or what to say so I just hold him and we lean back against the big granite slab. His skin is still cold from his having been outside and his knuckle bones look like they're going to come right through his skin. The TV makes a jolly noise behind us and the kids are giggling. A tomato has joined the asparagus now, and they're talking about the concept of promises with some grapes. Jack shudders and I think about promises too.

We go to Houston two days later, and the funeral Sandra gives her marriage takes much longer than the one I gave my childhood; her grief is long and aching. She weeps into our shoulders and tries to teach herself to sleep alone after almost thirty years beside the artificial safety and warmth of Sam's body. The shock is still rippling through her, but she knew, and so did Jack. For years, Sam's secret has been theirs too.

We're sitting in the little parlor room with Jack's siblings when he tells us that his dad has been unfaithful for years. He was sixteen when he came home from school and found Sandra curled up on the floor with the cordless phone, where she wept with her head on his lap. Apparently, a spurned woman had called to rattle off a list of Sam's conquests. It annihilated her, sent her straight to the ground. Jack says he stroked her hair and dabbed her tears away until Sam came home. Sam was sorry, he wanted to heal it, he and Sandra both did. Jack stayed quiet like they asked him to. He carried their shame obediently and silently from childhood to manhood. His siblings' faces stretch from anger to sorrow as he talks and we all grieve a death of our own: love isn't what we thought it was. I squeeze Jack's hand, but he doesn't squeeze back this time.

When we get back to Nashville, a few flakes of snow drift in a cold, still sky. There are late wedding presents sitting on the stoop, waiting to congratulate us and welcome us home: a set of flatware and a Crock-Pot from JCPenney in a big cardboard box. We bring them inside and go to bed.

The next morning, Jack is up before I am. He is showered and standing at the mirror, body wrapped in one of our many brand-new towels. He's looking at himself through a little cameo oval he's wiped into the steam.

"I don't want to be like him," he says.

"You're not," I tell him, but even I don't know how true it is, how much of who we are is sopped up from the people who made us and how much of our identity we get to construct on our own. We both stare at his reflection.

Over the next several months, his love for me is extraordinary, almost defiant. We spend as much time together as possible; I go on tour with him and he comes to youth group with me. We start to find the wholeness, the comfort, the belonging we were promised we'd find. Sam starts living with his girlfriend, Trish, while Sandra takes up hobbies she'll never maintain and tries to make a new life with the little bits of heart she has left. Marriage doesn't feel like the accomplishment it was last week; it feels like the beginning of a game we just found out we could lose. We play it very carefully.

8

Every Little Pill

Starbucks is not the best place in America to have a major health episode. It's too snugly wrapped up in its own contentment, its sugar cookies and free Wi-Fi, to notice anything remotely unpleasant. A person collapsing on the patio on a too-cold day in March can go completely undetected.

The pain is fierce and fast when it comes and it pins me to the ground. I am on my way to get a Power Punch from Smoothie King after grocery shopping, a task I've recently taken on because it makes Jack happy and it makes me feel like an actual adult. I pull into the strip mall and park. A welcome flash of afternoon sunlight jumps through the windshield and onto my cheeks.

A small pack of middle-school girls are hanging outside a nail salon, comparing identical pink toes and sucking the first coffee drinks of their lives down giant green straws. They remind me of the girls I teach at church, already drawn into the audition for womanhood, wondering if they're dressed okay or have the right kind of pretty to be loved by someone. The daffodils shooting out of the earth are enough of a promise for them to wear their flimsy spa flip-flops outside but they're stuffing their hands into the sleeves of their BeDazzled velveteen sweat suits. I smile big at them as I walk by and they smile back; they're delighted to have won the approval of a grown woman and I'm delighted that they think I am one.

I hop onto the curb and pull my hat down over my ears. The Starbucks is cuddled next to the Smoothie King and the entire block smells like muffins. I close my eyes and try to absorb it. I try to absorb everything about life right now. Jack and I have been married a year and a half and we're starting to understand each other; my middle brother, Tim, and Laura, whom we were right about him marrying, are having another baby; and the trees are covered in little green cocoons just waiting for the right day to burst open.

A big black bird squawks from the top of a streetlight. It scares me so bad my chest hurts. I wrench my head left toward the noise. Time is a sheet of blackness and everything changes.

It's quick and quiet, a lightning strike in my neck that shoots up into my head. The hollow smack of bone rings out as I fall to the sidewalk and the knees of my jeans become wet and warm with blood. Bolts of energy bounce through my skull and I slip into unconsciousness underneath a standing poster of a giant latte. I think about the muffins and have a dream I don't remember.

The *caw-caw* rings in my ears and my eyes fill with inky blotches as I start to wake up. I grab at the back of my neck and try to guess what the crap just happened to me.

Did I get shot? Run over? Pistol-whipped?

Is it a migraine? An aneurysm? Cancer?

Am I dead?

The pain is insane, throbbing and piercing and making my breath ragged. I lie there on the sidewalk, rolling my head from side to side.

Can anybody see me?

Anybody?

All the maybe-heroes are inside staring at their computers while a Norah Jones CD plays, singing to them about boat metaphors. It's just me, a village of wrought-iron furniture, and a Lhasa apso somebody left tied to a chair panting hot tuna breath into little floating balls of fog. I need a doctor. I need Jack. I need my daddy.

It takes a few minutes, but I feel clearheaded enough to sit up and lean against the window. An elderly man comes out of the shop with his drink. He struggles to push the slow-hissing door open and I wish I could help him. He ruffles the little dog on the head and smiles at me, completely unfazed by the fact that my shit is scattered everywhere and I look like I'm going to puke on myself. He walks over my tampons and pennies and hair ties and settles into a chair. Since I have a kind-of witness now, I feel safe enough to get up. I stumble to the safety of my Honda, turn the ignition, and bake in the car heat until I feel ready to drive. The migraine doesn't quit, so I drive slow. It follows me all the way home.

When I get back to our pretty yellow house I throw the door open so hard it rattles the glass in the windows. Jack is still emerging from a hard, heavy teenage sleep. He staggers out of our bedroom and knocks his shoulder on the doorjamb.

"Shit!" he says, pouting, and wiggles his feet half into his shoes to help with the groceries. He is too drowsy to notice my crazy eyes.

"Something's wrong!" I tell him. I lunge into his chest and press my head against the sour stink of his armpit. We sway backward.

I take a deep breath and say it again.

"Jack, something happened. Something's wrong with me."

He's bewildered. It won't sink in. His brown eyes are so wide that the crinkles in the corners disappear. It feels like the truest thing I've ever said but he can't tell if I'm joking.

"Babe, what are you talking about?" he asks.

He falls into the sofa cushions and Ellie jumps onto his balls with incredible accuracy. I sit beside him as he winces and grabs his crotch. We haven't faced a grown-up crisis of our own yet in the short, polite life we share together and he still doesn't know that I'm serious. He doesn't even know what "serious" would look like on me.

I tell him about the pain, the bolts of it, how it threw me down to the ground and left me with an insane, nerve-melting headache. I tell him about the little dog and the man and not being able to see properly. I tell him that I'm scared.

We don't know how to be anything other than nice to each other, so Jack covers me in his niceness. He leaps at the opportunity to comfort me, listening, rubbing my back, and giving me tiny quick kisses on the shoulder. He still can't understand; he just wants to make me not afraid anymore so that the rest of the day can be normal. He goes to the kitchen to get me a glass of water and stares into my eyes until the tears stop spilling over.

"I'm sure it was nothing. You'll feel better soon." He nudges a pair of aspirin across the glossiness of the coffee table.

No, I won't. You don't understand! I want to say it, but I don't, because I don't know how to be anything other than nice either.

There's an awful truth in me; it settles in my bones as Jack rubs his poor aching balls and Ellie wags her tail. It says that I'm never going to be the same, that life is never going to be the same. I don't tell him about it. Instead, I smile and pat his knee. I need him to believe in the easy thing we both signed up for, the glorious, uncomplicated future we designed together in my old apartment, with its vacations to Colorado and Christmas-tree shopping and pink-gummed babies that scoot across the floor. I need him to believe in it so that I believe in it too. Our harmless, happy little dreams are worth protecting. I spare him for today and try to trust in a sweet tomorrow.

The pain doesn't go away. Over the next few days, it happens again and again. It doesn't clock out at 5 p.m. to let me rest; it lusts after me, especially in the night. I can't sleep, and I start to dread the setting sun. The violet-spotted evening sky I used to love is just the opening act for wide-awake aloneness in the dark. I lie for hours playing jigsaw with pillows and throws, but there's no getting comfortable anymore. I beg for rest, I pray for it, but it never comes. I shake Jack sometimes, looking for him to rescue me, but all he can do is watch me lose the cruel night game.

"Shhhhhhh," he breathes, stepping just partway out of a deep sleep to speak to me.

I let him cover me up with his warm, clammy body; he almost has to hold me down. The sleep comes in the early morning and there's never enough of it. The truth in my bones speaks louder every day.

By April, I'm starting to miss work and my wonderful boss, Andy, gets worried. He calls to check in and I tell him over the phone what happened. Unlike Jack, he finds a hundred questions to ask me. He wants to know the exact location of pain, the exact location of the Starbucks, and if anybody in my family has ever suffered from anxiety. Andy's specialty is making people feel better, so he sets me up with a good Christian doctor from our church whose name sounds like that of a German Christmas cookie. Doctors scare me; they've scared me ever since I left Baton Rouge General with the brace fastened tight around my neck. I take the appointment though because right now, my body scares me more.

We go to the hospital on a Tuesday. I make Jack come with me because the smell of hand sanitizer and sight of scrubs return me to the bed, to the tubes, the pee bag. I think about the accident and I want to curl up into a ball and sob.

The office is on the fifth floor of a building called the "Doctor's Tower"; the name had to have been inspired by my actual worst nightmare. I hold my breath all the way up the elevator and plunk into a chair as soon as we arrive. Jack signs me in with his charming adolescent chicken scratch and says hi to the lady at the desk. We're a pair of *Sesame Street* opposites: He's bright, smiling, and sure that everything is fine; I am bracing myself for the worst under a cartoon rain cloud with Oscar the green trash puppet.

The exam room is papered in salmon-colored stripes and it smells like a Yankee Candle melted over isopropyl alcohol and sickness. Jack is standing guard beside me, squinting at a family portrait on the wall. It's an old picture, with gap-toothed children who are probably grown now and the golden kind of spouse and dog that every doctor probably has. The man who stands proudly beside them in the photo is a little bit fat and very happy underneath his giant red mustache. He walks in ten minutes later after a swift knock.

"You must be Ruthie." He smiles, cradling my hand in his and giving it a firm squeeze. He looks much older now than he was in the photo but still happy. He's shaved his giant red mustache and lost weight.

We sit across from each other, he on a short padded stool and I up high on an exam table spread with paper that crinkles underneath my butt. I am ready for him to fix me and Jack is ready for me to be fixed.

I tell him everything: about the accident in Louisiana, the Starbucks, the insomnia, the fear, the headaches, and the panic attacks. His expression remains friendly and professional the whole time, but I start to lose it. My voice shakes and snot drips down onto my sweater. Finally, I ask the question that I've been repeating to myself every five minutes since the day it happened:

"Am I gonna be okay?"

It comes out of me in a boogery sob. The doctor sighs.

I wonder if he knows that I *need* to be okay, that I need to be able to have babies and travel and dance. I need to know that the pillars of the rest of my life are still standing.

He hands a tissue to Jack, who hands it to me, and I blow my nose loudly and he tells us with as much certainty as he can muster that I'm going to be fine. He's amazed this hasn't happened before with my history; old traumas often leave intermittent pain behind when they leave and it's really nothing to worry about.

"We can manage it." He smiles, rocking back and forth on his wheelie stool.

Manage it. I repeat the words back to myself silently.

He writes me a prescription and orders some films. I fly out of the lab and into the fresh air when they're done. Everything is going to be okay.

In the coming weeks, the pain intensifies. I go to the doctor again. He refers me to another doctor and then another after that. They all stare perplexed at my scans. They point at a black spot at the top of my neck. When I ask about it, they tell me it's just the magnetism of the machine interacting with the wire in my spine.

They all have different suggestions but none of them has answers. They poke me with their cold, latex-covered hands; and they do more scans with more cutting-edge technology. In just three months, I have more pictures of the inside of me than the outside. I see a physical therapist named Janis who teaches me stretches, a healer named Steve who punctures my forehead with needles so delicate and hairlike that I can hardly see them. I try aquatic therapy at the YMCA, letting the liquid carry me across the pool while the Pussycat Dolls play in the background. When the doctors are out of ideas, my consolation prize is narcotic painkillers. Before long, I have a suitcase of them. This is what "managing it" is. I start back at work—we need the money—and though the pain doesn't dim, I get better at pretending. I put on a costume of my best, friendliest, most charming self for the people who deserve her.

The first time I take the hydrocodone I'm on a camping trip with fourteen-year-olds.

Every year, the church sends us on a retreat to Rock Island, Tennessee, with the youth group. We build pitiful fires with wet wood and talk about heaven and Christ and we eat s'mores. The site is buried in a forest on a shiny patch of limestone. Three foaming rivers meet there and burst into falls. It's the kind of beautiful, misty magic that takes your breath away but it's slippery and rocky and unforgiving on my body. I bring my pills along with me just in case. I still haven't felt brave enough to take them yet; the yellow warning labels scare me and I don't want to feel stoned, but having them feels like protection. Andy has his bear spray, I have my narcotics.

Jack comes with us this time, partly because he is worried about me and partly for the semi-spiritual nostalgia of it all. The gangly pines and songs about God are all like souvenirs of his childhood and he eats the entire experience up. He waves at me from across the tired flames, surrounded by a flock of needy teenage girls covered in bug repellent and blotches of self-tanner. I smile back at him as I load bottles of water into a cooler.

He is a good man.

Work has been punishing since the pain came, not just physically, but spiritually as well. It's hard to believe in Jesus's healing love when your body is betraying you. The kids ask big questions about faith and truth, and right now I'm asking them too often myself to offer any decent answers. I don't believe everything I hear in church. They say God is our father but the Bible feels feminine to me, like a mother. They say we're all broken but that feels so cruel, it feels wrong. They don't let women preach here and they don't accept gay people. Some of the white men who run our church don't seem anything like Jesus; they're hungry for cash and prejudiced. It's money for miracles and making sales of faith and collecting giving units. It doesn't feel good the way I want it to. I don't know what that means, but I can see God more clearly out here in the fresh air than I can in a giant stone building. God comes alive in the freckle-faced boys throwing footballs and climbing trees, he comes alive in the rushing water, he comes alive in Jack's big heavy arm on my shoulder. I walk over to him and we sit on a sideways log to watch a dance that we both know unfold: girls sitting on stumps with shirts knotted at the waist, frustrated and waiting to be discovered by boys who are too busy chasing each other to see them. Everything feels peaceful, but then the pain starts in.

The sun is at the absolute top of the sky when Andy, looking blistered and exhausted already, motions for us to round up the kids, twirling his finger like a middle-aged cattle rancher. We gather up the campers for the same hike we did last year, a soggy march that I know is sure to become a symbol for something biblical over hot dogs and thick gray smoke later on.

By the end of the first day, I am haggard and aching. Jack is in the boys' cabin. I'm alone in mine, exhausted and relieved to strip off my smile. Even if I'd wanted to do it, the pretending would be impossible right now because my neck is killing me and I have a migraine. I burned through my stash of Advil like it was trail mix on our hike along the river, and still I can hardly move. I need some relief. I pray and I wait, but nothing happens.

Standing in the tiny bathroom in my bra and panties with every busted inch of me on display, I survey my body in the mirror, shocked to not see it marred on the outside the way it is on the inside. I'm a human brochure for a healthier America: tall, thin, and, after twenty-five years of living in the South, perpetually cheerful. But I'm in agony and it is swirling right under the surface of half-decent skin and a pretty haircut. I wish I could wear the ugly naked pain on a T-shirt some days, so that it could announce itself and people would know not to expect too much. I feel like they expect so much. The tears arrive. I knew that they would. I set the pill bottle on the edge of the sink and size it up. I've never been hungrier for sleep, and the strange, scary tablets are all I have. I press down firmly and carefully, opening the lid for the first time and the chemical perfume hits me in the nose. I toss an oblong pill into the back of my mouth and swallow it with a palmful of water, stretching my neck like a goose to work it down to my belly.

That wasn't so bad.

I stuff myself into my bunk and wrap my body tightly in a flannel sleeping bag, just a giant plaid sausage of a woman. Then everything starts to melt.

The crickets' incessant chirps start to drawl out like telephone rings, long, lazy jingles that lull me into numbness. The medicine feels gentle and kind as it reasons with all the fucked-up parts of my body, my searing temples, my hunched shoulders, and the stabbing pain in my spine. It's like when my mom carried me downstairs at five years old and placed me into my sleeping daddy's bed, where I snuggled up next to him and let the shelter of his love hush my deepest, biggest fears. It rolls over me as warm bathwater does, from the top of my forehead to my toenails.

A half hour passes. An hour. The motion-sensor light flicks on outside the cabin and a swell of grave teenage shushing erupts somewhere outside in the dark. I hear the inevitable chaser of laughter and I know I should get up and send them back to their cabins. I don't, though. I let them run in the woods with their long, copper-colored legs and give their secret kisses knowing, as I feel the cool plastic of the pill bottle in my floppy hand, that you get to run in the woods for only so long before the young, pretty invincibility of fourteen wanders away. The drugs lurch into me, stronger now. They hold me down and force me into a peaceful, foggy sleep.

After we get home, I keep pretending for a while. I make our crisp white bed every morning, arranging our perfect grown-up pillows and wiping dust from the headboard. I light a candle that smells like old leather and take a long look at my work, a tidy little nest for tidy people. One day, I hike the mattress up on the edge of my thigh to make a perfect corner and my shoulders spasm. It's too much, I can't smile through it, I stop. I just can't do it anymore. I stop lying to myself, I stop with the pillows and the candles. I stop trying to make everything look perfect and neat. I give myself permission to get back in bed and I decide not to get up until the pain drains out of me. I drop my aching body onto the duvet and let my head sink heavy. I call in sick to the church and tuck myself in with reality TV and Cool Ranch Doritos. I wait there, I wait for weeks, but nothing happens. I go to work less and less, later and later, and I get more drugs, from more doctors, and I take them. The medicine feels like the only loving thing left for me.

Jack watches it unfold, but it is too big and adult for either of us to understand. He wants me to feel better and still believes in our sweet tomorrow. I pretend when I need to. I'm brave in front of our friends, I can dance and laugh and light up, but my limbs and the spirit holding them together collapse as soon as we're alone. Jack gets whatever is left of me after the show, the scraps. We stop having sex and he stops asking for it. Both of us are relieved to not have to navigate each other's bodies anymore. I move the pills to our bedside table next to a beautiful old bottle of perfume and I display them the way an old lady displays her collection of ceramic cats: my little pink Ambien with the perfect embossed letters; the see-through canisters of Lyrica; the melty plastic Cymbalta capsules that almost taste like sugar on my tongue; and the hydrocodone, my first love. They all stand proudly together, ready to serve me and love me in a way Jack can't, in a way he'll never understand. He does try, though.

One morning after walking the dog, he lies back down in the crumb-covered bed with me. He turns the lights down and watches a sweaty, shirtless man on *The Biggest Loser* step nervously toward a giant scale. He starts kissing me. I just lie there staring blankly at the TV. My eyes twitch a little as a beam of light hits me in the face. I didn't fall asleep until 5 a.m. and I am so starved for rest that my eyes have swollen to puffy slits. He stops with the kisses, gets up, and goes to the kitchen. He comes back with a box of Hefty bags.

"These are for the windows," he says, "so you can get some sleep."

Tenderly and lovingly, but with a sadness I can feel through my fog, he tacks them to the beautiful bay window, building me a fortress, helping me shut myself inside.

"Is this better?" he asks, begging for a sign of warmth from me.

I look at him, a sliver of hairy belly poking out from underneath his shirt as he flattens a piece of tape on the pane.

"Yes, it's perfect," I say, and it is.

It feels like the kindest, truest act of intimacy that has occurred in our lovely little bedroom. With gentleness and calmness, he helps me disappear. He was never able to figure out how I wanted him to love me in this room, but he knows what to do now.

He smiles, tucks the hair behind my ear, and goes to the bathroom for the first of a thousand glasses of water he'll bring to me.

Neither of us really knows it, but we have struck a new deal. We invite the pain into our marriage; we make space for it in our home and become a family of three. The man Jack expects to become at eighty-five, he becomes at twenty-three. He's the caregiver, picking up the laundry and ordering in. I'm the sick little wife. Pill after pill, season after season, I drift further away from him, from myself.

9

Harry Potter and the Little Black Spot

When something beloved breaks, people try to fix it. They panic, they spend the night on Google reading academic papers from the National Institutes of Health and watch tutorials on YouTube before YouTube can be trusted for anything other than cat videos. They leap down rabbit holes that are more like root systems, travel down winding corridors that sprout out in a hundred different directions, any of which might hold the answer, the method, the thing that makes it all better. When someone beloved is broken, however badly, whether they have the tools or not, those to whom that person is dear insist that she can be fixed. Over the next four years, everyone who loves me tries to make me whole again.

Jack tries to fix me first. He uses positive thinking and comforting words. When the Ambien doesn't work and my nerves are shot, he stays up with me as late as he can, forming my body into a crescent moon and pulling it into his. He moves the sweaty tuft of hair from around my ear and whispers that everything is going to be okay; he says it over and over again, falling asleep with the words still moving through his lips.

In the mornings, he wakes with me to the alarm bells on my iPhone: *Appointment!*

Therapy!

Take your medicine!

Our life becomes a series of scheduled experiments on me and Jack promises that today is the day, almost every day. He clings to the hope that *this* appointment, *this* medicine, *this* deep breath could be the healing, while I let hope slip like white sand through my fingers. He stands beside me for an entire year as I quit working and take up sickness full-time instead. He never complains about having to support us; he just keeps believing that I'll get better as we throw money at every possibility we can find, and as I slip away from myself to live life as a ghost covered up in our bedsheets. He loves that ghost the best he can, but it isn't enough. I can hardly feel his love, I can hardly feel anything.

The next year, after Jack tries to fix me, it's my mom's turn. I call her one morning when he's out on the road. I'm alone, and she knows she has to come see me the way some mothers, the best ones, can always tell when they're needed. She drives eight and a half hours from Louisiana to Nashville to mind me while I zombie-shuffle around the pretty yellow house with my big Ziploc bag full of medicine. Just like she did after the accident, she travels into the dark space with me as far and as fearlessly as she can. She rubs grapeseed oil into my shoulders in long, loving strokes the way Jack does and listens to me cry about the pain, the bills, and how badly I want to have children. She brews stinky herbal teas that are supposed to reduce inflammation and takes me to prolotherapy, an $800 orthopedic treatment that bullies the body into healing by sending it into trauma again. My mom sits in the corner of the room twisting the straps of her purse as the doctor injects my spine with a hundred little needles filled with sugar water. I can hear each one amplified through the speakers inside my head as it punctures my skin, *pop, hiss, groan,* and the serum rushes into me. After my mom goes back to St. Francisville, it's Katie's turn.

It's been three years since the pain began and Katie has watched all of it through her wise, soulful owl eyes. She and her husband, John, have two children now and live in the suburbs where the schools are good and the grass is short and green. She still loves Jesus and she still has the nubby-paged Bible she brought to Camp DeSoto. She's been praying for me, the congregants at her sweet little church have been praying for me, and one Sunday a woman there tells her about a famous faith healer coming through town, the kind who makes deaf people hear music and blind people see their reflections in the mirror for the first time. Katie knows I don't believe in miracles taking place on carpeted stages or in speaking in tongues. She knows that I'm angry at God, questioning him, that I have no desire to visit his house, since he refuses to come to mine. She also knows that I'm desperate, so she mentions it anyway. I call her the day of the service and ask her to come with me, which surprises both of us.

The church is a giant tower of blocks at the end of Music Row, an area of town filled with recording studios and record labels and country music managers, all busy plotting the takeover of pop radio. The healer is set to begin at 7 p.m. but the place is already wild when we walk in at six-fifteen. The sanctuary is like the trading floor of the New York Stock Exchange; too-loud background music thumps under our feet, and white men in suits wave their hands in the air. Everybody is dancing, but everyone is hearing different music; some people sway sweetly and others jog in place until they get big wet circles under their arms. Big pink and purple lights shine up from the ground, and tall, cross-shaped shadows stretch their limbs up to the ceiling. In big swirly cursive letters, projected text at the front of the room reads:

SO, DO NOT FEAR, FOR I AM WITH YOU; DO NOT BE DISMAYED, FOR I AM YOUR GOD. I WILL STRENGTHEN YOU AND HELP YOU; I WILL UPHOLD YOU WITH MY RIGHTEOUS RIGHT HAND. —ISAIAH 41:10

I glare at it and beseech it, believe in it and curse it all at the same time.

Where are you, God? Strengthen me. Help me.

Katie leads me up the steps to the balcony. We dodge believers who speak in tongues and stretch their arms toward the sky, begging the Heavenly Father to lift them. We pass people like me, broken and desperate, willing to sit through the magic show on the off chance that magic is real. We settle near the aisle in case I want to leave, and it begins.

A white-haired man with lily-pale skin and a headset microphone steps onto the stage. People scream for him, he's a Backstreet Boy, and the lights swirl and dance up and down the walls. At first he's soft-spoken, but he becomes so possessed by his own passion that his cheeks look sunburnt and fill with blood in the first five minutes. He talks about some of the great wonders God has delivered in his presence. This is when I really start to pay attention, when I try to find myself in his stories. There's the autistic teenager who started looking his mother in the eyes, the woman with a mysterious chest pain that the Lord lifted from her heart, the other woman with horrible psoriasis who now goes to the beach in a polka-dotted bikini.

The audience oooohs and ahhhhhs and amens and the lights swirl again.

I notice the man's son standing beside him; he speaks softly, a little awkwardly, and Katie tells me that he's hearing-impaired. He looks so tired. It's his job to play magician's assistant, to catch the falling bodies as they drop toward the ground, anointed. I see him take a big breath and I know the healing is about to begin. It's showtime.

A long line forms out the front door; people are anxious for their redemption, and an hour in, the stage is a battlefield, the healed lying still like the wounded with their arms crossed on their chests. The son is gentle with them, he's so careful as he arranges their limp appendages and puts his hands on their foreheads. One by one the bodies pop up, they raise their arms to the ceiling, and everybody cheers. Katie cheers. I take a deep breath, close my eyes, and hope for something extraordinary. The bright red preacher looks up, finds my eyes, and says, "Does anybody suffer from chronic back or neck pain?"

"She does!" Katie yells, grabbing onto my arm. "She does!"

Swirling lights and blurring and thumping music.

Instantly, the magician's assistant, the son, the gentle one who is hearing-impaired, is beside me and we're in the middle of the aisle under a hot white beam. He places his heavy hands on my shoulders. We stare into each other's eyes and I wonder how God decides who aches and who doesn't—why he stole part of this man's hearing and gave me pain. The man's eyes are olive-colored, steady and kind, and I don't look away from him while the rest of the room careens into a premature celebration of our healing.

Where is your miracle? I think at him silently.

I don't know, I imagine he thinks back, *but I have to believe.*

I have to believe too.

For a moment, as we hold on to each other, steady each other through the circus of color and music and faith, adrenaline resurrects hope. The man disappears as silently as he came to me and I feel lighter; I close my eyes as a giant mob of prayer forms around me and I dance my way into ecstasy. I wonder if this is finding Jesus. I wonder if God is finally paying attention. I wonder if I'm healed.

The days pass. The weeks pass and the miracle packs its bags and moves on just like the man and his son. I don't dance again for a long time. The seasons change and the skies darken to black wintry soot. Something in me darkens too. Jack is gone from the end of December to February. We talk less and less. I want him less and less. My caretaker, my confidant, my perfect codependent partner is a shih tzu poodle with an underbite, the only other heartbeat in the house. I talk to God less and less, want him less, and continue my slow unraveling from the church. All I want is relief, all I want is more medicine.

The pain wakes itself at dawn no matter when it goes to bed, and when I open my eyes, the first thing, the only thing I think of are the little canisters beside me. The sweetness of pills on my tongue is the only mercy, and though I don't abuse them, they abuse me, erase me. I become a robot fueled by shitty snack food and reality TV. I watch at least six episodes of *The Real Housewives of Orange County* a day. I disconnect from my own reality completely. The daily news looks like this:

Jo is trying to get a record deal.

Lauri gets engaged.

Slade dumps Jo.

Vicky drives her friends and family crazy.

I take up residence in their stucco-roofed subdivision by the ocean. I live in their stories so I don't have to live in my own.

When Jack comes home, he finds me listless, stoned, and frizzy-haired, carrying on an emotional affair with six women from Newport Beach, California. He doesn't know what to do so he calls his mom. Now it is Sandra's turn to fix me.

I go to Houston in March 2009, when the weather is just under eighty degrees and everything with blue petals is blooming. Jack is touring all over Texas with a big group of our most musical friends and I am meeting him there so that we can visit his family and try to be in love with each other again. When he's home, we go to therapy because I'm not communicating and we're not having sex and Jack is worried. I don't want to lose him, so when the therapist says we need to spend more time together I slap on a fentanyl patch, my newest strongest medication, and crunch my body into an economy seat on the airplane. I take a hydrocodone just as we take off and take a tingly nap the whole way there.

Miss Sandra picks me up from Love Field. I see her waving from the curb a quarter mile away in what is probably a new blouse she bought just to receive me in. She is the mom of three boys, so I'm an occasion for her, a glimpse of the daughter she always wondered about.

"Hiiiiiiii!" she sings prettily, and covers me up in her silky arms. "I've missed you so much!"

I climb into her SUV and she immediately presses a button that makes my seat sink slowly back as far as it can go. She wants to make sure I'm as comfortable as possible, and even though I feel ridiculous as I whir backward and away from her, I am grateful to be loved so well.

Sandra is happy now. She's married a nice man called Ron who is mad about her, and they live in a new beautiful home not far from the old beautiful home she lived in with Sam. As we drive she talks about her sons and Ron's kids and what we're having for dinner. She asks me about Nashville and about my family, and then, as the high-rises dissolve into the suburbs, she asks me about the pain. I tell her less than she already knows. Sleeping is hard, working is impossible, and insurance doesn't cover anything. She starts to ask a question but stops herself before the words come. In the same way my own mother, the best ones, just know how you need to be loved at any given moment, Sandra gifts me with a silence instead. She covers me in grace and understanding. I watch her shift in her seat and let out a long, quivery sigh, like it's all she can do to keep herself from jumping into my skin and carrying the pain for me.

"Did you remember to bring your films?" she chirps.

I did. I pat my bag. A fat manila envelope pokes out of the zipper pocket. Inside is every single image ever taken of my spine. Sandra has a doctor for me, just like everybody else does. She knows it might not work, but it's all set up and she'll pay for it, so it can't hurt. Trying to fix me is the only way anyone knows to love me right now. Letting them try is the only way I know to love them back.

The hospital is a stack of gray boxes in the middle of the city. We arrive early—Jack, Sandra, and me—after an evening of Texas brisket and watching lightning bugs fly in figure eights over the pool. My heart and backbone throb, kissing each other on the inside of my body as we skulk around the entryway and wait, white-coated strangers breezing past us like we're shrubs. My body remembers when it sees this place and I become allergic again, my throat itches and my hands sweat, and my breath is taken from me. Jack has walked me through dozens of these doorways before; his hand clutches mine and doesn't leave. It's routine, it's what we know, and all I need to do is hang on for thirty minutes.

The exam room is about the size of a changing stall at the Gap. The doctor stares at my films for a long time. He's tall, with a big mop of pigeon-colored hair, and stands with his hands on his hips like he's Christy Turlington.

"What's this?" he asks, squinting behind his glasses.

"My black spot."

That's what I call it. Nobody's given it a different name. He raises his eyebrows at the dark cloud at the base of my skull on all my films. I explain it to him the way it's been explained to me, nothing to be concerned about, it's just the wire interacting with the machine. He sighs and clicks his tongue.

"I can't help you properly until I find out what's underneath it."

He orders a set of X-rays that cost $50 and a different type of imaging that won't interact with the wire in my neck. I shake so hard when the tech injects dye into my veins that Sandra offers to buy me six months of PTSD therapy. It sounds like the most useful treatment anybody has suggested so far.

The call comes two days after my appointment and I let it go to voice mail. Jack and I are eating tacos together in Austin because it's easy to fall back in love with someone when you're eating tacos with them. The tacos are working, we're happy. The fentanyl patch is working too—it's strong. I can dance a little, snatch a glimpse of who Jack and I used to be together. I remember how hilarious he is and he remembers how much fun it is to be out at night with me.

I hand the phone to Jack to check the message while I get up to pee. He grabs my arm to stop me.

"Ruthie, this is Dr. Mills. You need to get back to Houston immediately."

We find out that the wire holding my spine together is poking into my brain stem. His voice is urgent. He's never seen this before.

"Everything is going to be okay," Jack sputters.

We leave our half-eaten tacos and everything else behind.

Back at Jack's brother's house just outside of town where we're staying, everybody panics, scurrying around, looking for something to do. Jack calls my parents; his brother John calls the insurance company; his wife, Lena, calls Sandra. I retreat, but Orange County isn't far enough away this time. I go upstairs and settle into the blinding pink of our five-year-old niece's bedroom. There are heaps of faded teddy bears, a neon-rainbow gymnastics outfit, and an owl decal the size of a Saint Bernard. I remember the joy of five and sit inside it for a moment, insulating myself with good memories for the rest of the evening. The next day, five years old doesn't feel far enough away, so while everyone else panics and fusses, I go to the bookstore and buy a half-off copy of *Harry Potter and the Sorcerer's Stone*, diving headfirst into Hogwarts to hang out with my friends Harry, Hermione, Ron, and Neville (who is the best one of all). I stay there, locking myself away in a make-believe world, which even with its spells and monsters feels safer than the one I'm from. By Rowling law, the dark is never as strong as the light and the evil can never unhinge the good. My heart aches for a simple justice like that.

We don't go back to Houston at all, even though we probably should. Jack tries to coax me, the families try, but I shut them all out. Miss Sandra overnights the films to my brothers in Baton Rouge and they take over. Tim is living a quiet life as St. Francisville's most beloved physician and Lile is living a loud one selling surgical equipment in the city; they call in every favor they can and set up consultations with the best orthopedic surgeons in the country. My parents talk over the possibilities, how they can help me, and what my life will look like if I need a wheelchair. I watch everybody spin and spin, worry and worry, but I stay still. Fear brings its own kind of paralysis.

After a few days, it's time for Jack to go back on the road with the band and for me to go back to Nashville with Harry Potter. I've been back just a week when Lile calls with the news: I'll need another surgery, another spinal fusion. He spoke with several doctors and the verdict was unanimous. I hold the phone to my ear for twenty minutes while his bellow of a voice goes on as he tries to be matter-of-fact, keep me calm, and reach me the way he's always been able to but suddenly can't.

"You're going to be just fine," he says.

I don't really hear him, I won't let myself. As soon as I hang up, I forget about Lile and my spine and the doctors, padding my brain with more magic spells and Quidditch tournaments. I keep my eyes squeezed shut as March becomes April, floating off, dis-associating, and letting everyone else deal with the business of me. With my eyes shut, though, there is so much that I miss.

I miss the panic and the pain, but I also miss the radical love. I miss the fear and uncertainty, but I also miss the belligerent faith of the ones who carry me, the wild courage they have to move forward when I can't move at all. I don't allow myself to witness the love that they pour over me; I just lie in my bed terrified, med-icated, paralyzed. I'm a ghost in the bedsheets.

10

More than God Can Count

My daddy's Amish friends live in Kentucky. They taught him how to plow with a mule and they broke his horses. When I was growing up, he would visit them every few months to watch the careful way they worked with their hands. They gave a gentle, loving touch to the most unforgiving labor: sanding lumber, wringing out their plain-colored laundry, butchering the animals they raised. He would bring them Honey Baked Hams, Tony Chachere's seasoning, and used books from his school. On very special trips, he would bring them turducken. The Amish go wild for turducken. In exchange, they sent him home with taut-skinned tomatoes; fresh, still-sweaty apple turnovers; and words about God and humanity that never, ever left his head. He drove them one town over to visit the doctor and go to Sam's Club and see their relatives who lived in simple, sturdy homes nearly identical to their own. He respected them. They were his best teachers and they loved him, flaws and all, just the way that we did. They became his family too.

My daddy's Amish friends baked yeast breads and sold vegetables by the side of the road, and they were loyal and humble and kind. They were the last people to see him alive.

My mom calls just after sunset. It is the middle of April 2009 and I'm leaving an Anthropologie store in the fancy part of town, just down the road from the slab of Starbucks sidewalk that changed everything. I have a new dress in a tissue paper–stuffed shopping bag, the air is the warmest it's been since winter, and my daddy is coming to see us tomorrow at 2 p.m. For the first time in a long time, I'm not thinking about surgery or pain or spines today. He's in Kentucky picking up a new donkey from his friends and wants to stop in on his way home. I don't know why he needs a donkey, but I laugh out loud when I think about him parking his livestock trailer beside our pretty yellow house in the middle of the iced coffees and MacBooks and beards that keep cropping up in our neighborhood. He left a voice mail yesterday and called me "baby girl." He sounded so excited to see me.

My phone buzzes like a wasp in my purse and the sound bounces off the cement beams of the quiet, covered parking lot that belongs to the Whole Foods one block over. I haul my body up into the too-tall seat of Jack's Expedition and I answer.

There are a lot of things my mom could say:

"Your daddy is going to be early."

"Your daddy is going to be late."

"Your daddy forgot to charge his phone again." There aren't a lot of places to charge your Motorola in Kentucky.

But instead, she says this:

"Your daddy fell. They found him unconscious at the bottom of a staircase. All we know is that they're taking him to Nashville, to Vanderbilt. He'll be there in two or three hours. Be ready to go see him then."

She doesn't really know what else to say because she doesn't really know what's happening. Nobody does. Tim's trying to get in touch with the doctors but the doctors are busy. She promises to keep me posted and I promise to pick up the phone. I stuff my things onto the passenger seat and drive.

Jack is at home when I get there; he's just gotten back from tour and we haven't even seen each other yet. He's wearing a shirt with a picture of a mountain on it and eating a messy, paper-wrapped bagel sandwich from the coffee shop across the street. He knows something is wrong as soon as he sees me. He hasn't seen a feeling on my face in weeks and suddenly, they're everywhere. The sandwich drops onto the floor from the table and he comes to me. I open my mouth to explain.

"Daddy . . . Daddy."

I can't get anything else out.

My body is shaking and I feel cold. The gravity of the not knowing pushes me into Jack's chest and he holds me, he hangs on to me as I go limp. We haven't been this close in weeks, not since we found out about the wire. After a few minutes, I tell him everything I know and we wait melted together on the couch for more news.

Tim calls an hour later. Outside the day has gotten dark but the sidewalks are still alive and gleeful like they were in the afternoon. Hipsters in too-tight jeans blow cigarette smoke from their noses and try to look aloof but I catch them through our front window looking up at the bright white, glow-in-the-dark dogwoods and smiling.

Don't they know what's happening in here? I ask myself as they stroll by grinning. *Don't they feel it?*

When the phone rings, I put it on speaker. Tim's using his doctor voice and I don't want to have to hear anything alone. Jack and I are on the couch but holding on to each other like we're in a lifeboat.

"Not good. Not good, Ru. It's time to go, he's not going to make it."

No. NOOOOOOOO! Nothing's meant to die in springtime. Poor sweet Dr. Tim, I can't imagine how many phone calls like this he's had to make. I can't imagine what it must be like to make that call to your own sister, to your family.

Before I can make a thought, we pack a bag. We drive past the chili-pepper lights of the Mexican restaurant with the three salsas that my daddy loves, the rough-looking grocery store he wishes I wouldn't shop at, and straight into the arms of the city that will hold him when he dies. We swerve and honk and accelerate under a big, bored moon that has seen everything before but on nights like this must wish it didn't have to. We get to Vanderbilt at 9 p.m.

They have a special room at the hospital for the people who are about to lose someone but it isn't really special at all. The walls are covered in lumpy, beige-colored wallpaper and there is an ivy plant that shivers under the AC vent the way everybody does in a hospital. We sit downstairs for an hour until a man with a sad, serious face comes for us. Two Amish people are already in the room when we get there, accompanied by their neighbor who drove them, Mr. Harold. He's a longtime friend of their Amish community and is also very close to my daddy. They're sitting at a conference table with their chins at their chests saying nothing at all, just staring at a box of tissues like it's a television set. There are enough chairs, the wheelie ones I love with whooshing hydraulic seats, but Jack and I collapse on the floor and drag our bodies to a corner. I hug my pillow into my chest, look up at the artless walls, and say, "Daddy, Papa, Dad. Daddy, Papa, Dad. Daddy, Papa, Dad."

If I call him the right way, maybe he'll come back to me.

A lady named Vicki comes to get me a few minutes later. She wears a turtleneck under her sky-colored scrubs because it's forty-four degrees inside. She has a soft, soothing voice that knows what it's doing, that sounds the way it should sound to do her job right. Her job isn't caring for my daddy, it's caring for us, leading us into the most sacred, horrible place in the world and coaching us to the other side.

"Follow me," she says.

She takes us down the hall past a pristine vending machine, full of Pringles and Nutter Butters, that I bet nobody has ever used before. People don't need movie concessions to watch this part of their story unfold. Jack holds my hand and swallows big as we walk, until we enter a very quiet room full of brain-damaged bodies behind walls of curtains and he has to let go from the shock of it.

"Take your time," she says, but there is no time left, it's already gone.

There is always something that can hurt more, a place to go inside yourself that you haven't explored, that you don't even know about. This morning when I woke up, I thought my pain was at a ten. I thought I was hurting as much as a person could, but when I pull back the curtain and see him there, it's an eighty-five, a 612, it's infinite. I'm being electrocuted from within all over again. The right side of his head is covered in a big, puffy bandage and he has a black eye making purple shimmer on his cheekbone. The left side of him looks complete, whole, normal. All his major injuries are concealed on the inside, just like mine were. They had to shave his mustache to fit the tube down his throat and it feels like an invasion, something I should have had to sign off on—and never would have. His tongue is out and he's wearing a gown covered with little diamond shapes that's too short for him, it hits just above the knee. He's sort of my daddy, but he's sort of something else, too, a magnificent shell.

I pat his hand the way he has always liked to pat mine.

"Pat, pat. Rub, rub. I love you, God loves you. I love you, God loves you. I love you more than God can count."

I look at his eyes and not in them, because they have forced them closed. He is more of a place than a person now, just a big empty house.

Katie and John show up, my surrogate family. Jack called them on the way when I was looking at the moon and wondering if it hated its job. Katie comes to me with her arms as wide as wings when we're back in the beige-colored room. She wraps me up, kisses me on the head, and lets me weep onto her shirt while she empties her cache of magical, limitless mom energy all over me. John talks politely to the Amish and then hugs Jack, who lets him do it even though I don't think he wants to. Jack doesn't want a set of arms pulling him further into the reality of today. They've come to take care of us because we are too broken to take care of each other, because we're suspended over grief, not sure when our tethers will be cut, and they don't want us to be alone when we fall in. Just past 2 a.m., Lile calls—they're five hours away.

I go back and forth from the room to my daddy every hour, from emptiness to emptiness. Katie and John and Jack come with me and they pray. Well, John prays because he's the best at it out of all of us. I try to be tender and together with my daddy just in case he can hear me but I fall apart into the different pieces of me within seconds every time I see his face.

I'm five years old, scraped knees and pouty lips and sobbing.

I'm fourteen and sullen and quiet.

I'm twenty-five and angry at God. I'm vengeful and I ask "Why?!" to nobody in particular.

I drape my body over his and I talk to him like he's still here.

When I'm back in the conference room, the motions of grief continue and Katie mothers me through all of it. Jack does the best he can: he rubs my back, blank-faced, pupils almost disappeared from the chocolate of his eyes. Jack doesn't hold me, but I understand why. Opening his arms would be an admission of defeat, an act of grief. It would mean he was accepting the unacceptable, that Lloyd Lindsey is gone, that he was gone before we even got here.

My family arrives in the morning around 7 a.m. My mom is frighteningly together, crying softly and gracefully into her hands. She says, "Thank you. Thank you. Thank you," very quietly, over and over again. My brothers tell me she was doing it the whole way here in the car, lying in the back seat. "Thank you. Thank you. Thank you."

None of us can understand the consuming gratitude of someone who has been in love for over thirty years. Even in death, she's indebted. She knows that gratitude is the purest form of healing; she learned that lesson too early in life, burying her mother at thirteen and bringing herself up.

Vicki comes back and takes us all down to him, a mama goose leading a string of her confused, dawdling babies. We hold his hands and kiss him and Tim says something meaningful that floats by me. Lile, the eldest, the rebel, the only one of us who truly felt the brunt of what happened to my daddy in Vietnam, whispers in his ear, "Don't take any of that bad shit with you. I love you so much."

We say our too-late goodbye to a man who has already left us; we touch him for the last time and wish he was touching us back.

A resident comes to meet with us in the big conference room and go over our options. They hand my mom an envelope with my daddy's things: his handkerchief, Swiss army watch, Saint Christopher medal, a pack of Certs, and some spare change.

"Is this all that's left of a life?" she whispers, and touches her lips.

The doctor shows us his films and tells us what we already know. He can't breathe on his own, he's not responding to stimuli, he's gone. It's over. He gives us fifteen seconds to let it sink in and begins to talk about harvesting the organs, the brilliant brain that held the brilliant mind, the hollow eleven ounces of the heart that nourished our family with love, the nearly blind eyes that hide behind his lids, they were useless but always full of joy. None of us can breathe. None of us know what he would have wanted or what we can bear. Lile speaks while we all realize at about the same time that we will never see my daddy wink at us from behind his glasses again.

"No. We can't send him in pieces. I want to be with him when he goes."

He's resolute.

We go down to see him one last time. A nurse waits silently behind the curtains until we're ready. Standing around him in a horseshoe, we enjoy the last bits of Lloyd Lindsey: the smell of his last breaths and the warmth of his skin. I tell him I love him. It's all I can say. When it's time, the nurse turns off the machine that was keeping the impostor in the bed alive, and just for a second, I look at him without the whirring chorus of the machine and I pretend he's napping. I could curl up next to him. Within a few minutes my daddy is gone. Everything is a blur, and I keep praying to wake up from this nightmare. It makes me feel sick to leave him.

A crowd of people have gathered to support us. I smile as big as I can at them, just like I used to do in second grade, even though I'm shattered. I let my body push me onward. We say goodbye to the little room near the Nutter Butters that will soon go to another family who just can't believe their loss, and we go. The Amish go back to Kentucky.

The city is bird-filled and beaming at us when we drive back to our pretty yellow house. The sidewalks in our neighborhood are busy again with rescue dogs and their overcaffeinated owners.

Don't they know that the best man in the world is gone? Don't they feel it?

I wait for the city to empty, for the sun to be snuffed out, for the world to stop, but it doesn't. It all just keeps moving forward.

Everybody stays with us for the night and we let ourselves be cared for. Friends show up with food so we don't have to worry about ordering pad thai, and they bring an air mattress that Jack blows up with an electric pump, and they pray for us. Miss Anna Klein, who works at Grace Episcopal in St. Francisville, finds my daddy a place to rest near a wrought-iron dove that hangs down from the boughs of a furry oak tree. It looks just like the one in the stained-glass window that we loved. Tim has friends who own a funeral home and they begin making plans for the service. Somebody from back home lends a private plane and arranges for all of us to fly home together. Nobody wants us to have to reschedule our grief, so they love on us. They show up. We don't have to do anything except survive and it's all we can do. Every spray of sunlight that settles on me that afternoon I silently pretend is him.

The airport is all flatness and big, barn-shaped hangars. We arrive there first thing the next morning and I'm so ready to go home, because being in St. Francisville is the closest I can get to my daddy now. Ellie wiggles in my lap as we park. She's allowed to come with us because people with private planes are allowed to bring their little dogs wherever they want to. She yips and her ears perk up; she has no idea what is happening. None of us do. We've gone straight from despair to the set of a Jay-Z video. Jack helps me out of the car and for the first time in two days, I notice my back hurting. I'm not numb anymore. I wish I was.

The pilot tells each of us that he's sorry for our loss as we climb the stairs, naked-faced and unwashed, wearing flannel pajama pants and dirty jeans. I imagine we're the least glamorous passengers that have ever flown with him before but he doesn't seem to mind. He gives me a bottle of water and I settle into the squishy leather seat. It's time to take my hydrocodone and almost time to take my antidepressant. I forget to brush my teeth but I never forget my medicine.

The plane goes up, up, up, and I float away from myself, tired and sick with sadness, wishing the pills still worked on me after four and a half years and that I could just be tingly and light for a moment. I stick my face right up to the window and Ellie smushes her nose against the glass. Life looks little and far away and I like it that way because it can just be a thing I hover above. My daddy and I never flew on a plane together but he would have loved it. He would have talked to me as we soared over the landscape, pointing out the big lakes and state parks.

"We're in Mississippi now, baby. Look at all of those gum trees!"

"The Native Americans used to call Lake Pontchartrain 'Wide Water' before the Europeans showed up and made a mess of things."

I can hear him. The harder I look, the closer I feel to him as we skirt the edges of where his new up-in-the-sky world meets ours. I stretch my eyes as wide as I can when I feel the drugs and the grief and the aching start to pull the lids down. I'm not ready to sleep.

Not yet. Don't go. I'm still listening, Daddy. Keep going.

I drift off with my hand in Jack's, head pressed against the window, listening to a quiet angel voice talk to me more about trees and the town where Muddy Waters was born.

11

Always Look Out
for the Little Guy

My daddy never wanted to get old. He watched his father get old, deteriorate, forget things. He would sit my granddad down in his living room chair and try to help him sort through his finances. They would have the exact same arguments every single week. Sometimes, my daddy had to write it down just to prove to him that the conversation had happened. Slowly, over years that just plodded along, he watched his papa fade into a cartoon, blank-faced, wrinkled, and confused. It broke his heart and it scared him.

On their way to a crawfish boil just before Easter Sunday, four days before his death, my daddy made my mom promise that if his mind left him like his father's did, if the boys he raised into men ever had to clean and dress him, she would take him out to the barn and let the mule kick him in the head. Two days after that, he woke up and told her about a dream he had about his old boys from Vietnam, the ones who never made it back. One day later, he went to Kentucky. There, he died of a brain injury and went home to rejoin his platoon.

He never wanted to be old, but he should have been older. He still had a lot of things to do here. So much life was left unfinished. He still had to meet my children, teach them about growing vegetables and watch them roll burly watermelons across the yard against the pink splatter of evening sky. He still had to take care of my mom, travel across America with her, and find the best hole-in-the-wall diner to get pie. He had to drink two thousand more cups of Community Coffee and read three thousand more books. He'd just voted for Obama. When he told me, he was sitting in his living room chair and his face lit up like a Christmas tree. He was so excited that America was changing, that maybe West Feliciana Parish could, too, and that the black kids at his school would have a president who looked like them. My daddy still had more work to do, more good to do. He still had to say goodbye. The architect of a family, the maker of all its best memories, should have had the chance, the dignity, of leaving the people he loved with a perfect, peaceful, expertly built monument of a goodbye. He never got to do that. He just left with no warning.

The Grace Church cemetery in St. Francisville sits at the corner of Ferdinand and Royal Streets. Fog rises up from the warm earth, through parakeet-green mosses, and into the loving arms of the oak trees, where sometimes it gets stuck until afternoon. Jackson Hall stands up proud in the middle of the headstones. This is where we celebrate everything in St. Francisville, including my daddy.

Everyone comes to the wake. The love for Lloyd Lindsey stretches up from the wet earth to the top of the sky, and old Grace, the grandest building I've ever known, is almost dwarfed by the ceremony of remembering my daddy. There are so many people, so many memories, so much to say that nobody thinks to stop and look up at the stained glass and spires. Inside Jackson Hall, it's elbow to elbow. People wait for hours sprawled across the squashy grass just to pay their respects: teenagers and white-haired ladies, the mayor, ex-cons, marines, total strangers, the boys who made it back from Vietnam, and cousins I pretend that I remember. The Amish are here. They chartered a fifteen-passenger van to drive them from Kentucky to Louisiana to help send their friend home. The high-heeled Ladies in Pearls are here, sinking inch by inch into the earth and ruining their best shoes while they wait. Cars sneak up the curbs and park illegally at foolish angles. The cops don't care; the rules don't matter today, because Lloyd Lindsey is gone, and even though he didn't get to build a goodbye for us, St. Francisville is building one for him.

My daddy was good but he wasn't humble. The sight of it all, the line snaking down the road outside the boundaries of town, would have had him feeling deliciously important. We never would have heard the end of it.

The casket is pine and still smells like the woodshop it came from at Angola Prison. The inmates crafted it for him by hand. My mom works at the museum there, and even though they normally make coffins only for people like Billy Graham, who won't die for almost ten more years, they make one for him. I hang my body over it all day, and the smells of sawdust and stain get into my clothes. Jack stands beside me and rubs my shoulders while my mom and my brothers bravely and graciously accept condolences from hundreds of people. The stories, the sweetness, the sorrow that drifts over to me make me miss him so much more.

I've never forgotten what he told me before school in the morning: "I love you so much, remember your manners, always look out for the little guy." But it's today, in a hall too small to contain the splendor of him, that I learn just how devoted he was to those words.

"He helped my mama move."

"He was the best teacher I ever had."

"Your daddy bought us a Christmas tree."

The mourners share with us for hours and hours. People we've never seen before, lives he changed but never spoke of.

"He helped pay my tuition."

"He helped me get a scholarship."

Lile wipes his eyes and Tim shakes his head. My mom looks deep into the eyes of every single person who greets her and gifts her with another memory. She says, "Thank you, thank you, thank you," with more sincerity, more truth than it's ever been spoken before.

"Mr. Lindsey sat with me while my husband was in the hospital."

"There's no way I would have graduated without him."

At the end of the day, I'm the last one to leave. Jack gently grabs for my hand.

"Babe, Ruthie, it's time to go home. The funeral is tomorrow, you can see him again tomorrow."

"Daddy . . ." I say it one more time, running my fingers along smooth marbled veins of the wood, and Jack leads me out the door.

The day we bury him isn't beautiful the way it should be. The rain works in long, boring shifts, tumbling fast from the smoky clouds and then slowing to a drizzle. The ground is gummy and everything smells like earthworms. The pallbearers wear his bow ties and the marines come in their dress blues. John and Katie come from Nashville. John sings "Give Me Jesus" and it reaches all the way up to the rafters. I smile the whole time, an enormous plastered Little Ruthie smile that makes my jaw creak. It's a weird time to smile, but maybe in this sadness if I look like a buoy, I can stop somebody else from drowning.

Jack peels me from the casket when it's time to sit down. I grin until my cheeks hurt.

My brothers speak during the service while I sit in the first pew on the right, irreparably broken and too skinny in an itchy black dress. I'm in awe of them and astounded that they can find words when I can barely breathe. Tim, who is quiet and somber but no more so than normal, recites Philippians 2 from memory; Lile makes a joke about our daddy getting chocolate pie on his angel wings and everyone laughs. Sobs float up past the white arches and get caught in the ceiling like fruit flies, buzzing and echoing and making beautiful, horrible, sad music. A few more people take turns standing up at the pulpit and preaching the gospel of Lloyd Lindsey, though nobody in the room needs evangelizing. I try to listen as they bring him back to life with their words, but I just keep staring at him in his big wooden box. The life of him and the loss of him sit side by side in front of me and I have never felt so much like I missed a step. My mom and I exchange shattered smiles, reading each other's thoughts, while the wild, ever-growing gang of nieces and nephews fidget in their church clothes and poke each other and don't understand why everyone is crying.

"He would love this," Jack says, squeezing my bony leg, trying so hard to make it better, to line it in silver.

"I know," I whisper. My cheeks are tired and shaky from making smiles I don't mean, but I make one more just for him. He's trying so hard to make it better.

When the service is over, we go outside. Long strips of sun stretch through clouds like spider legs as the pallbearers walk the casket across the twinkling green of the grass. They lower it beside a canoe-shaped hole in the ground and we all stand around and stare at the curves and knots of his new vessel. The sky suddenly turns deep golden and glorious and the air fills with the scent of *Magnolia fuscata*. It's time to say goodbye.

We all have our own ceremony for him. The marines raise their rifles to the sky and fire shots into the air; the Ladies in Pearls huddle together and cry; the kids wave their hands and blow him kisses. One of the pallbearers, John Roy, an old hunting pal, lifts a dog whistle from his pocket and puts it to his lips. The sound it produces, a series of short shrill rings, silences all of us. The marines jump in their boots and I see my mom smile for a minute. I can't hear it, but I can almost see *Thank you. Thank you. Thank you* on her lips.

"Come on, Buddy! Senator! Katie! Come on, Lou! . . ."

John Roy calls all the old bird dogs who died in years past to come welcome my daddy home, to join him in the field again.

". . . Choppy, Teacup, Belle."

He speaks, somehow, with my daddy's voice, and I wish he had a thousand dogs to call.

The drizzle stops. The sunlight is warm on me and on John Roy and on everybody and I hope that somewhere, it's warm on my daddy too. I stand there, close my eyes, and picture him surrounded by light and barking dogs, a garden for him to work and forest full of quail. I don't know how to say goodbye so I think it instead:

Goodbye, Daddy, I love you. You're my favorite, I'll never forget you.

Our freezer fills with food the way it always does in St. Francisville when something happens. Men come by to take care of the animals and sow seeds and the women check in, bring even more food, and tell us how beautiful the funeral was.

The day after the service, I go to see a neurologist in Baton Rouge. It's been a month since Houston. The only reason I agree to sit in a room with a doctor is because I don't have the energy to say no. Lile was able to arrange a surgical consult with one of his busiest doctor friends, and after losing my daddy, he's determined not to lose me too. Not even a speck of me.

Jack walks with me into the big, blond-brick tower and up to Dr. Paul's cold office. I wait, sullen, numb, and in fragments, for the better part of an hour, while Jack pats my hand and tells me he loves me.

When Dr. Paul finally comes, he comes at us quickly through the door in his scrubs. He shakes our hands and tells us he heard about my daddy, he's so sorry. I can tell that he really, truly is. He flicks on the light box that illuminates my films and starts right in. My daddy's nose and his chin and the cheekbone that he used to kiss before bed reach out to me from the bright white body parts. I cover my mouth when I see him there in me and I let Jack soak up what the doctor's saying because I can't absorb it.

The wire is there where the black spot used to be. It looks terrifying. It's stuck on top of the stegosaurus bumps of my spine and pokes just through the base of my head. I wonder how something so small could derail an entire human being. I hear my name but I don't respond to it. Words fly by me, past me, over me, and I just stare and wait to be done.

The doctor is staring between Jack and me. He doesn't really know who to talk to. I hear the word *paralyzed* and I'm jolted back, instantly terrified. Dr. Paul has my attention.

"The surgery needs to happen and it should happen soon. They need to remove the wire and perform a new spinal fusion. The risks are very high and we don't know how effective it will be, but it's your best option. As far as I can tell, this has never happened to anyone before, but if you don't get the surgery, you'll likely be paralyzed, and that could happen anytime. The longer we wait, the higher the possibility of permanent damage."

The fear and the missing my daddy and the injustice of living hit me all at once and I unravel. Jack shakes Dr. Paul's hand and we go.

"Fuck you! Fuck you! Fuck you!"

The screaming starts in the parking garage and the sounds swell and echo. I picture myself in a wheelchair, a vegetable who can't fit through the doorway with a husband who sticks around because he has to. We walk past kids with balloons and suspicious, slow-moving seniors who don't understand what they're seeing. Jack doesn't know what to do, so he grabs me firmly and supports my melting, furious body. He tries to get me to the car as quickly as possible while I cry and cry and scream.

"Fuck you! Fuck you! Fuck you!"

I've never said it out loud before. I say it to God, to anyone who's listening. I feel so far away from the God that my daddy taught me about, the one who is supposed to be good and just and loving. Where is all the good?

We get back to Lile's house and his wife, beautiful Libby, is standing on the stoop, waving her hand at a neighbor rolling by with her stroller. Libby and Lile are the fun couple on the street; theirs is the place where kids end up to play and parents end up to watch the LSU game. She touches my shoulder but I walk straight past her into the master bedroom and lie in their bed. The room where Lile sleeps, wherever it may be, has always felt safe to me. I dry-swallow an Ambien and look up at the light fixture.

Where is all the good?

That night, I can't sleep. I stand out in the yard at night the way I used to and smell the sweet air. I take the deep breaths my daddy taught me to and hope it will make me feel close to him, but my back aches as my lungs push into my bones. I raise my head to look for him in the sky, even though I'm scared that the next breath I take will be the one to break me, and I scan the constellations for a dog shape or a bow tie. I don't see him anywhere—I don't see good anywhere.

Show it to me.

My mom told me that the day my daddy died was the day he planned to tell me about selling the farm, his absolute everything, the earth he tilled with his hands, the magnolia tree, the hundreds of acres of playground I danced across growing up. He was going to sell it to pay for my surgery. The farm was his everything, and he was willing to let it go for me.

It's been a week. We're sitting around the Amish dining table in the farmhouse eating reheated sympathy gumbo, our last meal together before Jack and I go back to Nashville and life begins again.

"This came for you," my mom says.

I rip the envelope pitifully, like I'm splitting a log. I unfold a long piece of paper from the Bank of St. Francisville. It says RUTHIE MOORE MEDICAL FUND just below the letterhead. The account balance is $75,000.

My godfather, Mr. Carter, set it all up with my mom's blessing; they both knew it was what their boy would have wanted. The deposits are endless. There are dozens of individual contributions, some of $10, some of $4,000. As the days pass, Jack and I keep watching the balance grow from our computer in Nashville. I keep asking myself why, why these people, these strangers, would help me, and then I remember.

"He paid my college tuition."

"Your daddy fixed my roof."

"He bought our groceries."

"Mr. Lindsey gave me enough to get back on my feet."

"He believed in me."

He shows me, he reaches for me, he fills our world with his goodness just one more time.

The Ruthie Moore Medical Fund brings a glow to our pretty yellow house. Jack is renewed, resolved that everything will be okay. Even in my grief, I like seeing him happy, just knowing that he can be.

Our friends hear about the surgery and my daddy's death and the fund and they organize a benefit concert in June to help me, help us, with the healing. It's another party my daddy would have loved. The whole night I picture him walking around, shaking every hand he can find, and introducing himself: "Hi, I'm Ruthie's dad."

They raise $20,000 for me, and soon after, the surgery we could never afford, the one that my daddy wanted so badly to give to me, is paid for in full. It's the miracle, the testimony that everybody, Jack, my family, St. Francisville, needs to move forward. It isn't enough for me.

We have the money, I need the surgery, but I'm stuck. Fear lives where faith used to, and its roots have grown thick and knotty. Every day they don't open me up is another day I could laugh too hard, or change lanes too fast, or fall down a flight of stairs like my daddy did. Death feels so close since he left, moving with me through my day like a partner and keeping me aware that at least now I *can* move. If I have the surgery, nobody knows what will happen. Jack urges me gently toward the operating room with his hopeful brown eyes.

"No matter what, we'll get through it, babe."

But I don't really know that we will. I don't know if he can love me confined to my bed forever or wash my hair for me for the next forty years. I don't know if he's considered the future where I don't learn how to fish with him in the river or have his babies. For the next six months, he keeps nudging me, only bringing it up on the days the grief seems to have settled. My brothers press, too, getting as comfortable as they can in my daddy's shoes. They urge and they prod, but I put it off through fall and I put it off through winter. I meet with doctors and surgeons from across the country but make no decisions, flying over brown plains and lumps of mountain to waiting rooms and parking lots and tones of voice that are all the same. Some doctors want to fuse three vertebrae, other doctors want to fuse two. Two doctors want to fuse my neck to my skull so that I won't be able to turn my head without rotating my whole body. One doctor offers to do the whole thing for free. They're all eager to break new ground, to see something inside a person that nobody has seen before. Who wouldn't want to scrape away the surface of a new frontier? In fall, when I've sat in all the offices and gotten off all the airplanes, we decide on the Mayo Clinic in Minnesota. We schedule the surgery for April 2010. Mayo is the most expensive, over $130,000, but it's supposed to be the best.

Healing is a verb, a continuous motion. It's not a thing I can just reach out and grab, but I grasp away at whatever I can to hold me up through fear and through mourning that never quits. I keep moving, keep continuing, and keep trying to walk across the mucky fields of grief all the way through winter and into spring. I redecorate our house because there's no more Harry Potter left to read and I need something to get me through a full day from morning until night. I know I'll be spending a lot of time inside while I recover—if I recover—so I want it to feel good. Obsessively, I sink myself into project after project. I lie in bed looking for cheap internet deals on artwork and side tables. At the end of it all, my daddy is everywhere in the space I make for myself. He's in the brown-lacquered Amish furniture, the old history books, and the photographs.

When the house is done and I start to slip again, I reach out for something else to lift me. I have our friend Reid take pictures of each room and I submit them to the fancy design websites I fawn over. The pretty yellow house gets featured on *Apartment Therapy* and *Design*Sponge*; everyone we know—and plenty of people we don't—notices me. My story is big and public: it feels good to be noticed for something other than my pain. For a moment, I think about how proud my daddy would have been, instead of the fact that he's gone.

Friends tell me I'm talented and ask me to help with their spaces, and even though I need something else to grab onto, I'm still leading with fear. I can't ever bring myself to decorate for others. I go back to bed and look around at the beautiful shell I've built for myself, feeling my daddy's presence and absence in every corner.

12

What Screams the Loudest

The thing you hear first is what's screaming the loudest. I'm not sure if I made that up or not.

When I wake up from my spinal fusion at Mayo, the pain isn't just screaming, it's a siren. I can't see or hear or think—all I can do is survive from one second to the next.

Help me. Help me. Help me. This is certainly hell.

There are doctors and students and nurses in the recovery room, a little army of light-blue scrubs and latex gloves just for me. They busy themselves with tasks I don't understand, checking levels of things, writing words on big hanging bags of fluid and urine that look like what we used to hang on the porch to keep the mosquitoes away back home. They work, work, work all around me, testing my reflexes with a hammer the size of a toothbrush and shining a light in my eyes. Miraculously, I can move, but every movement is excruciating. Even breathing, inhaling and exhaling, hot air is a two-man saw pushing and pulling against my throat.

The more awake I am, the more awake I am to pain, to fear, to the loneliness of another sterile room full of strangers, and to my daddy being gone. My wild-animal eyes flick from side to side in my neck brace and I wonder if anybody will even try to meet them or if they'll just keep darting from task to task. I make an actual scream after a while, which I can barely get out. They just removed my breathing tube and the flesh is raw and swollen. The sound that comes from me is hoarse and not very loud, but it is impactful. The doctors move quicker, they juggle the bags, they try to fix it, fix me, but they can't. There is more quiet screaming. I'm a horror movie with the volume down.

"It's okay, hang on. Just hang on," they say, fumbling with the drip, adjusting the meds, checking the vitals, and wondering how much is too much and how much is just enough.

They up the morphine again but after years and years of "managing it," my body is bored with painkillers. There is no relief. There is no "enough."

"Just hang on, Ruthie," they say again. They're just a fuzzy talking cloud of people.

Hanging on is all I can do. I try, but I start to slip; my fingers uncurl from the edges of sanity, of safety, one at a time. I want my daddy so badly I can hardly bear it.

The surgery took more than eight hours. It lasted from about 7:45 a.m. to 4:30 in the afternoon. The doctors removed the parts of the wire that were sticking into my brain and left the rest. The other strands, which had welded themselves deep into the vertebrae, were too dangerous to fuss with. They re-fused C1, C2, and C3 with bone from my right hip, a little beam, and a bunch of titanium screws. I'm part skyscraper now. My family has been waiting all day in a little room with reclining chairs, bad geometric carpet, and free snacks. When you pay six figures for experimental spinal surgery, your family gets their Nutter Butters on the house. It's just shy of the anniversary of my daddy's death and none of us wants to be in a hospital again, no matter how many free Twinkies there are.

It is dark outside when they move me to recovery and my family can see me. They pumped me full of sedatives to keep me calm and I'm still sleepy, so I don't really see them back. Jack is the first one to come in. He walks from the door across the room to me and it takes a long time.

Left, stop. Right, stop. I make a little smile when I think it and my new neck brace creaks.

For the second time in my life, my head is half-shaved. It doesn't look any better now than it did the first time. My cheeks are swollen from the drugs; they puff out like Pillsbury crescent rolls and my eyes are glassy and bloodshot.

"Hey, babe," he says so softly.

I've been his patient for so long that seeing me sick and sore doesn't really faze him anymore. His brownie-batter eyes are gentle and teary; he hasn't had good sleep in far too long. He slips his hand under mine, slowly and carefully, nudging my fingers like Jenga blocks. He brings his lips down to my hand and kisses it; he doesn't want to hurt me. I don't want to hurt him either. Everything hinges on today, on a few screws, some doctors, and a bit of metal. I wonder if it worked, if I'm all better now. I wonder if we've been delivered back to our happy, hopeful dreams.

The others follow him in. I hear Lile before I see him, and he tries to make me laugh straightaway. Tim can't find his way out of doctor mode and politely needles the nurse about spinal fluid leakage and vital signs. Aunt Raven brings my mom to me. She's here, but she really isn't. There are two smears of blush on her cheeks and she's smiling, but even in my stupor I know how sad she is, to be back here in a place like this, to see another part of her soul in a diamond-print gown, hooked up to monitors and machines. If she could, she would travel into the darkness with me, I know it. She can't, though. She could barely make it through the wintry sludge in the hospital parking lot to the front door. There are too many memories, too many shadows in her own world for her to find a way into mine.

Lile finds *Benjamin Button* on the TV in the corner of the room and they all watch me eat a glob of green Jell-O that I can hardly control on my spoon. When a nurse comes in to check my incision, my brothers and Raven go to the Marriott Courtyard across the street for the night. Jack and my mom fall asleep on a pair of foam-stuffed couches. I stay half-awake, kind of stoned, enviously watching Brad Pitt go from an old aching man to a little boy.

In the morning, the sedation wears off completely. The screams are so loud that Lile hears *me* first for once, all the way from the elevator. My mom and Jack are white-faced and waiting in the hall while the doctor checks me. Lile bursts by them and through the door. The safety of his face is the only respite.

"What's wrong?" he asks the doctor, and the two of them talk while I concentrate on breathing and beg my body to pass out.

Before the surgery, I told the doctors that my pain was at a ten, but there's always something that can hurt more. This is immeasurable.

Lile's phone rings. It rings again.

"Sorry," he says, as the doctor continues talking.

A 911 text from his mother-in-law comes through. Then another one. He wants to throw his phone out the window, but instead he disappears into the hall.

When he returns, the doctor has finished and gone on to peek behind other bandages. My mom and Jack are on either side of me, holding on to my hands.

"Baby, Libby's daddy was in an accident."

Lile is still stoic but the words are a struggle.

"Libby!"

It's one of the first words I can say clearly. I try to sit up. They all tell me to rest.

"I need to go back home but everything's going to be okay."

He has to go home, I want him to, but I also need him so badly. He feels like the only shelter I have left.

Everything's going to be okay, everything's going to be okay. I put it on repeat.

Three days in, my sight goes black and blotchy, my brain feels like it's being rolled over again and again like dough. It's the worst headache of my life. I'm screaming and writhing as much as I can in the big creaky brace. Jack runs out of the room to find the doctor and comes back with a light-blue army for me. The doctor checks my bandage while I make my sad-coyote sounds.

"Shit," somebody says.

I'm leaking spinal fluid; my neck brace is soaked with it. They need to reroute the fluid to control the migraines, so they schedule a lumbar drain at 2 p.m. Jack doesn't know what that is but he nods up and down furiously like he's been thinking it all along. I will be awake for the procedure, which is my worst nightmare brought to life. They're going to puncture my spinal column.

A resident comes into my room that afternoon carrying a metal tray just like the one they carry my lunch on. Instead of turkey sandwiches and apples, there are tools wrapped in plastic, lidocaine gel, and a needle the size of a Bic pen. I give my consent; our eyes meet for just a second. It seems like we're both terrified of what's about to happen. A team of sturdy-looking nurses come in to help move me. It feels violent, like a beating, when they curl me onto my side and ask me to arch my back like a cat. I scream and cry and try to claw my skin off.

"Please! No!"

They keep curling me and I can feel the life drain out of me. Jack and my mom leave the room, they have to. They've seen enough—probably too much—and they can't bear it anymore. The nurses put their backs into it, they start to sweat and tremble for what's about to come. The resident wipes my back and begins.

The very edge of the needle meets my skin, just tickles it, and then plunges into me. It groans through the tissue, severing fiber after fiber, and the pain is a warning bell that goes forever. He pushes it deeper and I want to throw up.

I don't know what's happening. I can hear him breathing and grunting. He stabs again and again.

"Please! Stop! You need to stop!"

I can't hang on anymore, I'm slipping, falling, screaming, crying, I'm going away. The nurses hold me tighter.

He tries again, the needle pops twice, once through my skin and then deep inside, to a chamber of my body that I didn't know I had. I'm in the jaws of something. There's a hammer or something pounding the needle in farther.

"Not quite," he says.

He tries once more, twice more, three times more.

"Just hang on, sweetie," the nurses say, their faces hot and clammy. "You're doing great."

No more. Take me to the barn. Let the mule kick me.

God abandons me in this room. My daddy abandons me. He gores me for what feels like twenty whole minutes.

The sky gets dark early, and mercifully, the resident gives up. They call in a new doctor, who takes me to an operating room and uses a tiny camera to place the drain. It takes about three minutes. Once it's inserted, they say they fixed the problem, that the damage has been prevented, but I've never felt so damaged. In spirit, I'll never be the same.

I'm discharged from Mayo after just one week. I walk out of the hospital in my big creaky neck brace, one hand in Jack's, the other clutching a big paper bag filled with pills, many different types of medicine, more than I've ever been on before. Tucked into my right palm, tucked into Jack's hand, is the wire they pulled from my neck. They let me keep it as a memento, a pair of Mickey Mouse ears.

We sit in the hotel room that night and examine the wire. We have to, as so much of the history of us is tangled up in it that we can't look away. It's thicker than we thought it would be—more menacing. Jack looks at me hopefully. He brings me my water and kisses my head. "It's over now, babe."

I stand in the Marriott bathroom the next morning before we leave with the wire in my hands. I touch it and smell it and turn it in all directions. I hold it up to the light and try to decide how many inches long it is. I don't know what to do with it. It's a strange artifact, a part of me. I want to back over it with the car and display it on the mantel all at once. I toss it in the little mesh wastebasket next to the toilet but I can't leave it there for long. I wrap it in toilet paper, shove it in my bag, and bring it home with us.

We prayed that when I woke up from surgery I would be able to move, and I can. We assumed that if I could move, I would move forward, life would move forward, but it can't and it doesn't. We prayed for a new beginning but we forgot that beginnings are work. They're nasty, struggling, treacherous things. The pain is still excruciating and the little wire never really loses its power over me, over us. The hinge we hung it all on breaks. We slide backward into the mud. We built an entire future around an event we had no control over. Complete recovery was the only bet we placed, and we needed the win. Over and over again, this brand of hope forms the basis of so much suffering.

"Just hang on," the doctors say, but we lose our grip.

When we get home, we wait for the new beginning we were hoping for. I wait for the pain to go away; Jack waits for the girl he married to arrive. He stays home with me as long as he can, bringing me breakfast in bed and making sure that I have enough pillows. People show up with dinner and cards and flowers every three days, Jack heats up lasagna after lasagna. He waits and he waits.

For a month, he walks me proudly around the block in my giant neck brace and short, bushy LPGA haircut. They told us the walking would make it better, would help me heal, so we walk for miles, we walk like our lives depend on it, but nothing changes. When I become less of a spectacle, the homemade chicken and dumplings stop arriving on the porch, the friends stop coming by, our mothers come for their visits and they go back home. Everything is quiet and we're left in the pretty yellow house to try to find each other again, but we just can't seem to do it. After six weeks the pain transforms into an awful searing, a constant burn. It feels like being bitten by red ants and I need my medicine all the time just to survive hour to hour. I panic when I can't find the right pill at the right time and Jack has to calm me, he has to reason with me like the toddler we don't have together. He gets frustrated and I don't blame him: our new beginning has already begun, but the story is the exact same. He leaves for tour and though he'd never say it, I'm sure he's glad to be gone.

I walk almost fanatically while he travels. They said it would make me better. I take my medicine fanatically. They said it would make me better too. I follow every instruction precisely and I wait for the chapter to end, for the redemption I'm owed to come to me. I walk past the perfect pine fence that encircles our property, a gift the Amish built to honor my daddy. I put my hands on it every day, trying to soak up all of him that I can. I walk down the street to the little garlicky restaurant at happy hour to watch pairs of girlfriends talk with their hands and splash cranberry juice and vodka on the sidewalk. Maybe if I just keep walking, I'll find my way out?

"Just give it time," Jack says chirpily on the phone from Milwaukee or Madison or Mars.

"I love you, babe."

I don't have any more time. We don't have any more time. Come home.

There are a hundred things I feel but I don't say, don't feel that I can say anymore.

"I love you too."

Four months go by, four months of walking and waiting and walking and waiting and trying so hard to make the new beginning begin. I get a fresh set of X-rays done to send to Mayo. I see my daddy's nose again and his chin again and I miss him so much I have to grab onto the little composite office desk to hold myself up.

The orthopedic surgeon calls on a Thursday. I'm walking the sidewalks through a summer sun shower. Jack is away somewhere—San Antonio or San Diego or Saturn. It is too hot out and the shingles are steaming rainbow mist from their blackness but I keep walking anyway, I keep the promise I made. I do the work, I take the medicine. I get myself ready to be whole.

"Good news, Ruthie!" The doctor's voice sounds like happy music. "Your films look wonderful. You've healed beautifully."

Healed.

I reach back at my neck to pick at another piece of dead skin above the incision.

"You can begin weaning off the brace and go on to do most exercises and activities."

Healed.

I reach my porch and sit down on the steps. I suck in a deep breath and the sour B.O. smell of the plastic brace hits my nose.

Healed? But how?

My treatment is complete. They have done everything they could do.

"I'm still in a ton of pain . . ." I start in.

"You can continue to manage any pain. . . ."

Manage it.

I've been here before. I remember the very first doctor who wrote the very first prescription during our very first year of marriage. He told me we could manage it, but managing pain isn't the same as healing it. This hurting and medicating and needing to lie down can't be fixed, only covered up.

I get off the phone, go inside, and take the neck brace off for a few hours. I keep following instructions; they are the last instructions I get and I cling to them. I let my skin soak up the air-conditioning for a few hours and I put the giant plastic prop in my closet next to the hats.

I lie on the beautiful bed in the beautiful room I designed for myself, for my new beautiful beginning, and I think about promises. The quiet bargains we make between ourselves and the invisible things we think hold the power to turn hope into change.

If you smile big, people will like you.

If you lose God, he'll come find you.

If you take your medicine, it will make you better.

"Just hang on," they say, my mom and Jack and the church and the hospital.

But what happens when you don't have anything left to hold on to?

13

C. Diff Is Not a Rapper

I was six years old when the baby came to visit us. He had bright pink cheeks and fleshy, star-shaped hands and he reached for me every time I entered the room. I sat on the couch and his mom laid him on my chest, the flutter under my ribs against the beat of his busy little heart making the most perfect, awkward jazz. I lay with him until time got lost, while his parents talked to mine, trying to figure out why it all felt so sacred, why the weight of his body felt like the answer to a question I hadn't come up with yet. I knew in that moment as he laughed at me for trying to find bones under his puffy, cloud-shaped thighs, as I drank in the sweet and sour of his skin, that I was meant to be a mother. Every single year from then on, I asked my mom for a baby for Christmas. As a child, I knew it was something that I would need to be whole as a woman.

At thirty-two years old, falling to pieces in the darkest dark, I still believe it.

It takes me a while to realize that our marriage is falling to pieces too. I can hardly see it withering as I wither alongside it. It happens slowly and I miss things. I miss the moment Jack starts touching me the way a doctor touches a patient, I miss the moment I stop aching for him when he's away, I miss the page on which I begin to write him out of my story. After the brace is off and I finish my treatment, after we know what I am and what our life will be—chronic, everlasting pain—I go back to my bed and Jack goes back to work. His heaviness returns and I don't even think to help him; passion dulls to fondness, fondness to friendliness, friendliness becomes duty. He checks out, and I let him go. The distance between us becomes so great and impassable that we're just hazy dot people on each other's horizon. I see his fuzzy dot waving at mine but I can't tell if it means hello or goodbye.

We try working on it. We go to our therapist to fix the communication things. I buy an on-sale vibrator from the Hustler Hollywood store to fix the sex things. I throw him a birthday party and bake him a cake from a box, but it isn't enough. How could it be? For years, when he was busy taking care of my pain, he had his own hurt, and with nobody to tend to it, it grew wild. He looks at me, at us, through a shadowy, pain-filled lens of his own. There's only one thing I can think of that could close the gap.

We've both always wanted a family: pure, unspoiled, sustaining love that fed us both well growing up. We've never used protection. Every single month since we married at St. John's, the gunmetal-gray church on Old Laurel Hill Road, I've secretly hoped I would get pregnant. It hasn't happened yet and I don't know why. I've gone to hundreds of baby showers, and at every single one, I've ached for my own bundle of helium-filled pink and blue balloons. All of Jack's friends have kids. They play on little soccer teams with Day-Glo jerseys; they go on fishing trips; they get little toy drum kits and tap away together. I know that he's ached for all of it, to be loved that way. A child, the biology of his parts and mine together, the science, is all we have left to give to each other.

One morning when the sky is just waking up in long strands of light, I think about the baby with the cloud thighs and I wake Jack, who's snoring beside me, face pressed down into the pillow.

"Let's have a baby. Let's really try. Let's be intentional."

He blinks at me a few times and he agrees. We force a new chapter.

Baby-making sex is not a steamy, against-the-wall thing, it's an unromantic, clinical, at-just-the-right-time thing. I learn about ovulation and periods and buy a plastic barrel of prenatal vitamins from Walgreens. I ask my doctors which medicines I'm allowed to take during pregnancy and I imagine decorating a nursery, which will be pretty but not dainty. We have official baby-making sex three times a month on the days that babies are supposed to like to be made the most, and afterward, I lie in bed with a pillow under my butt and my legs stuck up in the air.

"Do you think it worked?" Jack asks, leaning across the bed and looking at my belly. I laugh at him, we both laugh. It feels so good.

Often I think about what our baby will be like, long, lean body and little Tic Tac toes, bright blue eyes that will turn to mahogany just like her daddy's, a mop of wet-looking dark hair that will fall out onto her crib sheet and give her silly bald patches. Having a thing we can yearn for together feels like stepping into a warm bath. I imagine the weight of her on my chest; I imagine her on Jack's chest. I imagine all the ways she will heal me, heal us.

Every month for half a year, my period comes. The excitement of the trying wears off. We step out of the warm bath and all the little bits of hope have been sloughed off. The baby that was supposed to heal us begins to destroy us. I sit on the couch and cry as the cramps radiate around my middle like an inner tube, mingling with the pain, the awful burning that goes up and down my spine. Jack sits with me on the twenty-eighth day of each month and rubs the big red splotch on my back that the heating pad leaves behind. He brings me my water and cares for a brand-new affliction: infertility. Like always, he does the best that he can. He says the things he's supposed to:

"It will happen when it's meant to happen."

"Don't worry, the worrying isn't good for you."

"I love you. We could adopt."

None of it helps me. The only one that can help is the baby.

Some days, I blame him. I get angry. I tell him he's drinking too much, that he's not trying as hard as I'm trying and it isn't fair. He shuts down, shakes his head, and walks away from me. Our ocean grows a little deeper, a little wider, and our dots take a few steps inland. I start to blame my own body too. I look at it naked in the mirror. It's a shitty, broken-down, malfunctioning machine with a tampon string hanging out and I just fucking hate it. I hate the way the light settles on it, I hate the hip bones that still stick out like a child's, I hate it for all the ways it's failed me. I decide to take it to a new mechanic.

Miss Carol is an ob-gyn in Baton Rouge. She delivered my brothers' babies and she's friends with my mom. She works in a giant women's health complex where you can go to get liposuction or chemotherapy or a green smoothie. She's called me "sugar" for as long as I can remember. Miss Carol wants to help us have a baby.

We visit her in fall 2011, when the first morning frost of the year is lying heavy on the ground. She sticks an ultrasound wand covered with freezing-cold lube into me to look at my uterus, and she presses down hard on my belly. A screen beside the bed lights up, and Jack and I both stare into my black, empty womb. It's the first time I've ever seen it, its sad little moon crater. She presses more and moves her wand and decides that everything looks good. Jack looks at me and smiles—we're not used to hearing doctors say that anything about me looks good. I see hope on his face again. Then she sends Jack with a stack of magazines to a windowless room, where he ejaculates into a little cup. They test his sperm and it looks good too.

Miss Carol has a plan.

"We'll try a few months of Clomid. It should help to stimulate ovulation and make it easier for you to conceive," she says.

She hands me a foil packet of pills and a big instruction booklet, and walks us to the door.

"You're gonna do great, sugar." She smiles and squeezes my shoulders in her hands.

Again, the answer is another drug, another medicine, another bunch of tablets that will sit next to my bed with the rest of my collection.

We try the baby pills for three months, but they don't work. We try a type of artificial insemination called IUI, but it doesn't work either. The space between us grows even deeper and wider. My desperation grows deeper and wider. The burning in my body is as constant as my pulse, and some days I don't even know if I could care for the child that I've dreamed of for so many years, but I don't want to give up on her. Motherhood feels like the only thing left for me. When Miss Carol says there's one more thing that we can try before IVF, I decide to do it.

My mom drives me to the hospital in Baton Rouge early in the morning. The roads are empty and peaceful and the blue of the sky is swallowed by a sunrise that stretches all the way around in violets and magentas and strips of orange. I'm having surgery today. Miss Carol thinks I have something called endometriosis, which means that the uterus lining doesn't grow where it's supposed to, making it harder to get pregnant. The only way to be sure I have it is to go in through my tummy and check. When I schedule the surgery, Jack's in Australia touring with a famous vegetarian pop star and won't be home for weeks. He doesn't want me to do it, sit under the gray sky of another frigid forty-four-degree hospital and be put to sleep. I suspect that he doesn't really want me to have the baby anymore either, but he's too nice to say it.

My mom pulls into a spot right next to the entrance, another sliding glass door in another imposing brown building, and I take a deep, shuddering breath, preparing myself to revisit Mayo and Baton Rouge General and Vanderbilt and every doctor's office I've ever been to all over again. Jack calls on FaceTime just as I'm getting ready to walk through a set of doors without him for the first time.

"Are you sure you want to do this, babe?"

His face is a concerned, pixelated jigsaw. I look at him frozen on the phone, oceans away from me. Then I think about the baby and how she could heal me, how she could heal us.

"Of course. I'll be fine."

And, clinging onto my mom, I walk inside.

When I wake up from surgery, I know that something's wrong. Hairs on my stomach pull up from my skin as I breathe; there's a gluey little bandage, but it's not where it's supposed to be. I'm in a room surrounded by curtains, just like the one my daddy was in when he died, with an IV taped to the top of my hand. My arms are blotchy and cold. I stretch them out and wish there was someone to grab onto, Jack or my daddy or Lile. The nurse in the corner is busy picking her nails. She looks at me like I'm a thing when she notices my big, open eyes, and lazily, she pages Miss Carol.

My mom's face is a beacon when she peeks past my curtain a few minutes later. Miss Carol is with her, as is an older, quiet-looking man.

"Do you remember Dr. Fife?" Miss Carol asks, looking excitedly over at the man, then to me and back again. He has the kindest eyes and a big gray Santa beard. I'm so confused. She goes on.

"Sugar, when we went to look at your uterus, we noticed that your appendix was about to burst. We brought Dr. Fife in to perform an emergency appendectomy."

The man waves at me like we're old friends, but I've never seen him before—he's a total stranger. He smiles.

"Ruthie, I removed your spleen in 1996 after the car wreck. I recognized you."

I recognized you.

He recognized me splayed out on a table, eyes closed, absent, big broken husk of a body on display. He probably saw the scars he made and, like everyone else seems to, he probably felt pity. It's been a long time since I've been recognized for anything other than pain.

It's been such a long time since I've been anything other than a thing to pity, a collection of sickness and scars. My mom and

Miss Carol and Dr. Fife stand outside the curtain and talk about my care. They laugh about the smallness of the world and how funny life is and what he's been up to but I stay silent. I can't stop thinking about what he must have felt when he saw me there on his table again.

I recognized you.

But really, I wasn't there. My soul was sedated, on holiday from the dreary place it lives.

I recognized you.

I wasn't even there. I haven't been for a long time.

I stay in the hospital for the night. I don't have endometriosis. Miss Carol says that everything looks perfect and that it's only a matter of time. The part of the hospital I'm in feels more like a museum at night, quiet, calm, and echoey. The nurses who come by speak softly to me, and even though I want to, I can't sleep. It keeps playing in my head, over and over again:

I recognized you. It consumes me.

Staring up at the ceiling, I whisper-chant it. It swirls inside my head and follows me all the way back to Nashville. I wonder what the doctor saw when he looked at me: a collection of scars, a victim, a lost cause, a burden. Those are the things that I see. The child who loved her daddy, who danced barefoot until dinner and felt safe in her own skin is unrecognizable now. She's gone.

The stomach pains start in the middle of the night. I've been home for two weeks and Jack is here. In the morning he's leaving for the southeast leg of a US tour and I'm supposed to go with him. I stumble to the bathroom. I don't have any time to be slow and careful with my body, so my right side is in flames when I crank my limbs out of bed and drag myself across the floor. I sit on the toilet and everything drains from my body. Dr. Fife told me that the antibiotics might make me nauseous, but this is different, it's food poisoning on steroids, it's fucking hell. Jack snores away in the bedroom. I could wake him, he would want me to, but I'm tired of being his responsibility. I want to be his wife again. My body spasms for two hours until the sun comes up.

"Babe," Jack says in the actual morning. He's about to leave and I'm not going with him because I'm shitting my brains out. "Do you want me to call someone?"

"No! It's just a bug. I'll be fine. I can fly and meet you."

The air in the house smells like sickness, the slow-death perfume of a nursing home or mortuary. I stick my head out from behind the bathroom door and meet Jack's brown-gravy eyes one more time. I have the fan going so loud that I have to shout.

"Really, I'm fine," I promise. But I'm not.

For the first week, I tell myself it's the flu. I have diarrhea thirty times a day, and the longest I sleep is for an hour-long stretch on the bathroom floor. I buy a pack of enormous incontinence pads for myself, longing to buy diapers for a baby instead. They hardly fit under my jeans, and I crinkle like a tissue paper–stuffed gift bag when I walk. I have to wear them, though, I'm leaking and it won't stop. I tell myself it's nothing, just a bug. I'll get better soon and then I'll get pregnant. The second week, I'm still leaking, still waiting to get better. A photographer we know named Sara calls. She saw the pictures of the pretty yellow house on *Design*Sponge* and wants to use it to shoot the cover and artwork for Taylor Swift's new album. I wonder if she can hear my pad crinkling through the phone. I'm tired of saying no to things, of being a patient, another thing to care for like a potted plant or a gerbil, so I say yes. My body begs me not to. I have to double over to get the words out but I do. Sara says she's excited. I call Jack and he's excited too.

The morning of the shoot, I stumble around hunched over and I light five different scented candles to cover up the smell of the bathroom. The crew arrives at 10 a.m. with their bright lights and hard black gear cases. I smile big at them and show them around while my face turns green. When Taylor Swift arrives, I smile really big at her too. I try to stay and help while they get ready but my back is sweating. They're playing amazing music, Paula Abdul and Mariah Carey, but it all sounds like nonsense to me. I look down at my stomach throbbing through my shirt and I clench my butt cheeks together. My pad crinkles again.

"Y'all, is there anything else I can do?" I get extra Southern when I try too hard.

I wait for them to respond. Their faces are blank and their brains are busy with other things. The dampness under my arms turns to wetness.

Jesus God Universe Dumbledore!

I don't even know who I'm talking to up there anymore. I'm gripping onto the edge of my favorite chair and grinning maniacally.

"Nah, we're all good." I don't even know who says it.

I waddle-run across the street to the little coffee shop, where I stay squatted over the toilet almost all day. My good friend Taylor leaves in the evening, and I go back home and squat for another full week.

I'm not old, but I do know what it feels like to be close to the end of life. It feels like I've been perched on the edge of that pool for years. One night, I get very close to diving in.

I'm curled up in bed, it's past eleven, and I'm in anguish. My stomach is so bloated I feel like it's going to pop out of my skin, and even though I've been trying hard to take care of myself, I just can't. I need help. I call my old church friend Debbie. She's the first one in my phone and she has a teenage daughter, so I know she'll answer when her phone rings on a Friday night. She comes right over.

Her eyes are huge when she sees me.

"Oh Ruthie," she whispers. Skin hangs from my face like old theater curtains. I try to make a smile for her but she doesn't smile back. I'm skinny. My pants fall down when she helps me stand and she pulls them up for me.

"I'm sorry, I'm sorry, I'm sorry," I cry over and over again.

She guides my salty, wet body to the car and drives to the hospital, to another brown-brick building, with another sliding glass door. They diagnose me with *C. diff* quickly. *C. diff* is not a rapper—it's a bacterial infection. It normally occurs in senior citizens, in the weak and sickly, in people dipping their toes in the end of life. It makes your colon swell to the size of a Butterball and you shit like a garden hose on full blast until you die or it goes away. I likely caught it in the hospital while trying to make my body ready for a baby. They give me another pill, more medicine to make it better.

I recognized you. It plays and it plays and it plays.

I go back home with my instructions: isolate, medicate, disappear. Don't infect anybody else. Keep all of it to yourself, your sickness, your decay, you could hurt someone. I stop sleeping. I can't. I just stare into the brokenness. I can see it now, a big, open, throbbing blackness in the floor. The shame is all over me, it's all I can feel. My brain swirls around in busy, blurry circles. I think about Jack, the boy I met, married, and ruined. I think about the baby that doesn't exist. I think about the God who never listens. I'm not sure he exists, either. I stay up for four days, adrenaline slamming my heart against my chest.

"I recognized you." I start to say it out loud.

I decide not to tell Jack what is happening. I tell him about the infection but I don't tell him what's really happening, that something snapped in me, that I haven't slept or showered in days. I don't tell him that our bed is full of garbage and that I keep forgetting to flush the toilet, that more than anything, I want to go to sleep and never ever wake up. I talk too quickly on the phone, round and round and round, wild and manic like an auctioneer, but he doesn't notice or he doesn't care. Our friends keep bringing me things I don't want, pity casseroles, Gatorade, grocery store flowers, but I keep them all at a distance. They watch me, worried, and I understand. I can step outside of myself and see it: I'm a hyper, thin, pet-store puppy in a glass box panting and pawing around in the sawdust.

Laura calls a lot. My mom calls a lot but I'm always too busy swirling to talk. When I finally do pick up, all that comes out of my mouth is gibberish. My mind gives in to the brokenness of my body. My mom drives to Nashville through the night and takes me back home. I go back to the place where I began.

14

Red Ants

Red ants are an invasive species. They don't belong in the spaces they colonize and once they arrive, they're nearly impossible to get rid of. They'll eat anything: watermelon, earthworms, flesh. If it's too big, the army works together to break it down. They're aggressive, crawling up the body like it's a tree trunk, anchoring themselves to the skin and stinging repeatedly in vertical swarms. The more times they sting a person, the worse the reaction will be. It can take your breath away. Red ants aren't just pests, they're predators.

It's July and I'm back in St. Francisville. The outside air shimmers like hot oil above the old gravel road, and the horizon quivers and sways in front of me. I get lost in the ripples, the mirage I grew up wondering about but forgot to find an explanation for. Big, blind jade-colored beetles fly in circles above Lake Rosemound, bumping into each other and falling into the dirt. They make this place buzz from May until Christmas. I sink my toes into the scratchy brown sand of a beach no bigger than home plate. My granddaddy built this lake; it's right on Lindsey Lane. I learned to swim here and made fishing poles out of sticks and bright colored yarn. Tim's girls are splashing and screeching the way I used to, but it's too loud for me today and I can't concentrate. Tim and Laura and my mom are at a picnic table drinking fizzy water and I know I should go join them but my body is stuck, I don't know how to direct it anymore, how to put one foot in front of the other without an escort. Nobody's coming to get me, so I just wait, counting birds in the sky. I get stuck at six and start again.

"RUTHIE!"

My name is coming at me from a faraway place. I close my eyes and listen to water sloshing gently around. I start counting the birds again. *One, two, three, four, four . . .*

"Ruthie, *move*! They're all over you!"

My shoulders go pink with heat; the sun is in the middle of the sky and the little black birds put on a show for me. They're diving shadows dropping down into water, one, two, three, three, three . . .

"MOVE!"

Tim runs toward me, making a burst of tawny dust, and points down at my right leg.

There are red ants all over me, from my ankle to my knee. They're cinnamon colored and frantic, crawling up and down, navigating the kneecap and the tendons and the too-long leg hair. Hundreds of little teeth sink into my skin, but I've been hurting for so long I hardly even notice. I'm totally disembodied. Trauma sends an invitation to go away and I accept it. I've left my home. My body is vacant and my soul is buried so deep under so many layers of pain and trauma, I hardly even know it's there.

Tim looks at me. His polo shirt is soaked between the shoulder blades and has become untucked from the waistband of his khakis. I don't know what I'm supposed to do. He shows me how to swat at them, then leads me down to the edge of the shore and tells me to sit down in the shallow, cold, murmuring water. The girls stop playing and just stare at me until my mom fishes me out. The birds are all gone now.

"Come on, let's go home now," she gently sings.

She holds my hand and leads me back past the brick-colored dune. My brother sad-smiles at me and pushes his glasses up his nose.

Nobody knows what to do with me. We all go back to the farmhouse for dinner, my mom's tomato pie, and I rub ointment onto the bumpy, fire-red ant bites. Ellie licks it off right away. Tim prays before we eat but I can hardly hear him. I can hardly hear anything over the thoughts that go round and round and round. Laura nudges me every few minutes.

"Ruthie, sweet girl, take a bite."

Tim and Laura were supposed to be on vacation in North Carolina but they turned around when my mom called and told them she was going to get me. Laura wept, she'd called me so many times but I just didn't pick up. She was worried that my mom wouldn't make it to Nashville in time.

After dinner, she leads me to my bed, where I will lie awake all night panicking. She pulls the covers up and reads to me. The girls are outside playing and screeching again. I can hear my mom and Tim talking downstairs.

"What is she on? What did they give her?"

"Where's Jack?"

"Lord Jesus, how do we help?"

Jack's in Australia and I don't know when he's coming back. He might've told me or he might not have, but I can't remember. We don't talk on the phone anymore and both of us are thankful to have literal oceans in between us to blame the distance on. Laura recites me something from the Bible with her hands on her chest and I wonder where God is. She seems to find him in every passage, but I can't see him anywhere.

In the morning, my mom takes me with her on errands. I'm not allowed to be alone and she doesn't like to be alone either. She still doesn't know what to do in a world without my daddy, so she does most of the same things every day. We go into St. Francisville for groceries and dry cleaning and to visit my daddy's resting place. She shows me the smooth ashen stone they placed at his head, the dove that sits above his beautiful, holy name. I put my hands on it and try to feel him, but it's just cold stone on my fingers. My mom tries to feel him too. She's been trying to feel him ever since he left.

A little list written on old stationery is her guide through the motions of the day. She clings to it so she doesn't have to think about him too much. We zip from place to place. She drives too slow and talks at me too much but I like being buckled in next to her because it feels safe. We roll past the places I used to play: my high school, Mr. Carter's house, the street that leads to Hardwood, and Sonny's Pizza. The radio station buzzes in and out. I begin to regret the funeral I gave to my childhood. I would give anything just to dig it up and jump back in.

The drugstore is the first stop—I need my prescriptions. The drugs don't make me feel better anymore but I get sick if I don't take them. When we left, I was almost out of my fentanyl patches and my Cymbalta and the Ambien that doesn't work anymore.

The little door chime that used to love to jingle is old and flat. It clangs at me when I lean my shoulder into the door, and slowly, just barely, I open it wide enough to walk through. The inside of the store is too bright and too white and the music is bad. I grab for my mom's hand and she leads me through the corridors of razor blades and two-for-one loofahs to the pharmacy counter.

"Ask him about my patch," I beg her. "Please."

The man in the white jacket is patient with us. My mom rifles through my purse to find the papers she needs and he raises his eyebrows up high when he reads about all the medicines. My mom obediently asks a question about the patch, keeping her voice low like he's a drug dealer. He sighs at her and shakes his head.

"Maaaaaaaarsha!!!!!!"

Suddenly, a woman with swatches of pink lipstick on her forearm runs up to greet my mom.

"Baaaaarbara!"

They hug and gab and their jewelry jangles. They talk, not about anything important, just so that they can stretch their lonely, widowed voices out. The woman asks how the kids are doing and my mom smiles.

"Oh, you know, busy as always."

They laugh. I'm not sure either of them knows why or cares.

"Everybody's doing so wonderfully," she goes on. "Tim and Laura just got back from vacation, and Lile and Libby are at the beach with Parks. They sent the older boys to camp. Annnnnd my sweet Ruthie is here with me for a little visit."

I'm sitting in a vinyl chair next to a blood pressure cuff. She points at me and smiles. I have dog breath and I haven't washed my hair in weeks. The right side of my mouth twitches as I try to make a smile for them and the woman pelican gulps and tries not to look too shocked.

The pharmacist hands me a paper bag filled with narcotics and tells me he can't get the patch without an in-state prescription. I start to shake. That's the one I need the most.

"Well," my mom says, "we better get moving! Good to see you, Barbie."

She leads me slowly to the door. I bump into the Ricolas on the way out and hear them topple to the floor.

"It's okay, Ru," she says, patting my arm.

It's not okay, though, and people know that. When something happens in St. Francisville and people don't know how to show up, they gossip instead. Everybody knows that Ruthie Moore is unwell and it isn't the kind of thing you can fix with a covered dish or good pie. I've been here for only a day, but I can feel the news, the pity swelling across town.

My mom loves me as best she can, half-broken herself. She pretends that everything is fine and she clutches her little list, hoping that it can fix both of us. When people whisper and look, she just smiles big and says, "I love having my girl home."

The shame swallows me in one bite.

I go to stay with Lile and Libby the next day. I need to be near Lile—he's the closest thing left to my daddy. My mom willingly hands me over, she knows she can't mother me right now, and with three young boys, Lib is an expert in mothering. She met Lile in college at LSU and he couldn't have dreamed her better, springy chestnut hair and root-beer brown eyes like Jack's. She makes him laugh harder than I've ever heard him, and she gave him a trio of sports-obsessed sons. She didn't grow up with much, but though she learned to love on little, she learned to love well.

When she hears that I'm coming to stay she gives Little Lile's room a hasty feminine makeover. There's a floral comforter on the bed when I arrive and a vacation-scented candle called Aloha Orchid that's been burning for hours to get rid of the peewee-football smell. Even though the whole family are raving mad fans and it pains her to do so, she untacks his LSU posters because she knows I'm too fragile to fall asleep with fifteen cartoon tiger mascots watching me.

There's a newly formed village of framed photos on the dresser across from the bed, one of Jack lifting the veil from my face at our wedding, another of the nieces and nephews at Christmas, and my favorite, a rumpled old picture of my family at Perdido Key in the '80s. I'm about ten, my skin is the color of pralines, and I have long spindly foal legs. My daddy is supposed to be smiling at the camera but he's smiling at me instead. I move it over to sit right next to me by the bed. *Daddy.* I wonder what he would think of me now.

Lile is harder on me than Libby is. He's straightforward and makes sure that every word he says to me sinks in. He makes me get out of bed every day, hands me a towel and points me toward the shower. He calls Jack on the phone and tries to fix my marriage, when he sees that I'm alone in it. He steps up without hesitation as a brother, husband, father, and friend. He makes doctor's appointments and forces me to come and eat dinner at the knotty pine table. Their youngest, four-year-old Parks, sits beside me, and Lile fathers both of us through the simplest things.

"Ruthie, try the black-eyed peas. Parks, drink your milk."

"Ru, look at me when I'm talking to you. Parks, go wash your hands."

It's humiliating and necessary. I don't have anywhere else to go.

In a week, the color they got at the beach has drained from their faces. I can see them aging by the hour and it kills me. The shame is killing me.

The days are hard but the nights, the nights are fucking terrible. They're purgatorial. At 7:30 p.m. Libby puts Parks and Rhodes down to sleep. She reads them a story about a blue truck, holds them long enough to drink in the smell of toothpaste and little boy, and turns out the light. A few hours later, Lile starts to nod off watching ESPN highlights and stumbles off to bed, where Libby waits with her nose in a magazine. It isn't a sudden departure but it always feels that way. I'm alone. Everything is dark, everything is quiet, the floorboards stop creaking, the faucets stop running. I am all that's left in the world, pitiful, wounded, awake.

Lile sets an alarm for 1 a.m. to check on me. Even though I

see him there standing over the couch and talking, I can't speak. I don't even remember how. I just lie there, big white eyes peeled open and pointed at a television that isn't even on. He pats my hand and I watch him grieve me. It's like I'm already gone.

I did this to you. I let you down. I'm so sorry. I can never say it, but it blows by in my swirl of thoughts every thirty seconds. He's always been so proud of me, but now he can't even trust me to survive a night on the couch.

I make my way to Little Lile's room and crawl underneath the covers by 2 a.m. I read my daddy's Bible. I pray, I go through the motions of Christianity and wait for salvation. Then, I notice the old purple Tiger clock on the dresser, *tick-tick-tick-tick-tick-tick.*

The countdown begins. My blood goes through me in surges; every vein is choked, then released. Hot, roiling adrenaline shrinks my lungs into a pair of tiny brown raisins and I can't breathe. I try to get comfortable but there is no comfort—the red ants are always there under my skin and in my belly, marching up and down. I kick and flail and Libby's nice flowered blanket falls on the floor. I scratch at myself, at imaginary, nervous itches I invent. I take my clothes off and hug the pillows into my chest. Another Ambien, I take just one more and I wonder why it isn't working, why none of it ever works. I'm a failure, I'm a cripple, I'm a burden. *How did I get here?*

Then the shame that chases me during the day closes its mouth around my neck and speaks to me.

Look at yourself, it says. *What a waste of breath! Your daddy is so ashamed.*

My eyes shut and I beg for something beautiful. I think about Laura Treppendahl.

Laura, Laura, Laura.

It's very late when I begin to feel her with me. I keep my eyes closed, put my hands on my chest, and make a little extra space for her. I can see her dewy angel skin and her big eyes and her skinny shoulders that always shake like maracas when she laughs. I think about how kind she was and how sad I am that she's dead. She would be doing good in the world; no amount of pain could contain her joy. No amount of pain could sour her heart or cool her devotion.

She should be here, not me.

She should be here, not me.

She should be here, not me.

I repeat it obsessively in my head. It never stops.

Around 3 a.m., I try my daddy's Bible again. It's still filled with the scrambled teeny words I can't make any sense of. There's a billowing under my ribs and I beg again for something beautiful, something that will save me. I see my daddy.

Daddy, Daddy, Daddy.

If God is so good, why did he take you? Why did he take Laura? Why did he spill such ugliness over his masterwork? Why did he leave me here to suck the life out of everyone I love? I'm so ashamed, so irreparable. How do I find my way?

I can see my daddy plowing the garden. I can smell the hot manure and feel the steam rising off Amos the mule. There's a pink 6 a.m. sun behind them as they go up and down. He's smiling at me, so big, the only way he knew how. He speaks to me without words.

"Don't you see it? Look at the sky."

The exhaustion sets in and he fades off somewhere. I try singing "Give Me Jesus" in my head but I can't remember the words. The room is quiet and the red ants march faster now; my body is angry and weary from so many sleepless nights. The scrape of English muffins flying out of the toaster comes and my eyes are still wide open. Lile knocks.

"Ru, get up, come have some breakfast with us."

And I go through the motions again.

I see Dr. Wyatt on a Tuesday. It's after six in the evening and I've been in Baton Rouge for ten days. Dr. Wyatt specializes in pain management and her waitlist is eight months long. Someone who lives one street over from Lile and Libby does her billing and calls in a favor, so she stays later than normal just to see me. The office is freezing. I haven't slept in three weeks and I'm shaking, all nerves and Freon. Libby's right beside me. I can tell that I'm hurting her, rubbing her arm so hard it could catch on fire, but she doesn't say anything; she just pats my hand and shushes me. Lile is on the other side of the room, bouncing his heels up and down.

Dr. Wyatt doesn't make us wait long—she's already gone through my records and she knows what she's dealing with: the concern is written all over her face. She enters the room, a talking blur of skin and doctor jacket and orange cat–colored hair, and I can feel her looking in my eyes and trying to find me. She huffs fast and hard out of her nostrils and the rush of hot nose air makes me blink.

"Ruthie." She grabs my hand. "I'm not even concerned about the narcotics. The first thing we need to do is get you some sleep. You can't find relief without rest."

Lile and Libby become ten years younger in an instant. There's a plan, there's hope.

Dr. Wyatt prescribes me something strong for anxiety. She's bewildered when she looks at my meds, seven different kinds in staggering doses.

"How did this happen?" She shakes her head but doesn't expect any of us to answer.

I wouldn't even know what to say if I could form words properly. I just did what I was told. I took the pills they told me to take and waited to feel better but it was too many, too much, the kind of cocktail given to a terminal cancer patient entering hospice, a little something to make death taste better. All it ever did for me was make life taste worse.

When we get back to the house Tim and my mom are there drinking sweet tea. Little Lile is back from camp and he's playing football all over the tan couch cushions in the living room with his brothers. Their little bodies fly into old thigh-shaped pillows and make the fabric bunch and ripple. They want to talk to me.

I sink into the beige furniture, square in the center of the people who love me. Tim and Laura, dressed as though they're going to a luncheon for the Horticultural Society; Lile and Lib, dressed as though they're going to a tailgate party; and my mom, looking as beautiful as ever and lonely without my daddy sitting next to her.

"Baby, there are places you can go to get help. . . ."

I'm not sure who says it. I'm too tired to find the face that the voice belongs to and too overwhelmed by the gravity of the words to respond to them. I don't want to be sent away.

I travel from them while they talk, back to my childhood. Back then, all I ever wanted was to be the center of it all, to be seen and doted on, but today, in the middle, holding every eye and heart in the room, all I want is to disappear. The distance between

Jack and me is big, but the one between who I am and who I long to return to being is bigger.

They go on, avoiding words like *hospital* and *pain clinic*, and I half listen, terrified not only of the hospital, but of that great distance and what other people would think. Little Ruthie who danced on the porch, dripping with promise, can no longer function without pain pills and had to be shipped off like a bad dog. I won't let it happen.

Tim pulls me back into the reality and asks me a question I haven't been able to answer in a long time.

"Ruthie, do you want to live?"

I nod, bug eyes still wide and empty. I'm surprised I still know how.

"Then, babe, you need to get out of bed and begin. You can lie there and hurt or you can live your life and hurt. You can love people and experience things and hurt at the same time."

They decide to let me stay, to let me try to get better at home. I promise them that I'll start making changes, weaning myself off the drugs, if they give me another chance. I don't know if it's remotely possible, but I commit to it and they don't bring it up again. That night, I take my anxiety medicine and I sleep for the first time in twenty-one days. Dreams come: I'm six years old, dancing across the wide green lawn, smacking jade-colored beetles as I twirl, letting the sun be my stage light. My foot hits a dusty hill and the red ants come. They sink their teeth into me. There are dozens. I swat them away and I keep on dancing.

15

Operation Sunset

In life, sometimes we make lists of things. We make them so that we don't forget, so that we know what it is we're supposed to be doing. I have no idea what I'm supposed to be doing. I forget how many times a day to brush my teeth and when people eat lunch and what to do in the blocks of time stuck between meals. So I source the information of what a regular day entails from the life happening around me at Lile and Lib's. Showers are in the morning, lunch occurs around noon, the cleaning up of books and toys falls in the evening. I write everything down in a list and I cling to it just like my mom clings to hers. I call it "Day":

> *8:00 a.m. Get out of bed. Do NOT get back in until it's dark outside.*
> *8:05 a.m. Brush teeth.*
> *8:10 a.m. Make bed.*
> *8:15 a.m. Toast*

It's 8 a.m. I'm four minutes into weaning myself off the drugs and I have felt every second go by. The sun finds its way through the curtains and into the margins of my little Walgreens notebook, the kind that divides your life with flimsy plastic partitions. I pick it up from the bedside, stare at my schedule, and the warmth from outside waves at me through the window. It's time to begin.

The rest of the house is awake. Rubbery kid shoes squeak on the floor and water rushes through the pipes. The door opens and closes, letting hot breaths of Louisiana air whoosh their way inside. Lile, Lib, and the wild little boys they made all know what to do with a chunk of morning, but I'm so nervous about surviving the time between tasks that I can hardly stomach the sound of them all living so expertly. To me, it all looks impossible, like acrobatics. Little Lile's Tiger clock ticks at me while I walk to the bathroom and wait by the sink until exactly 8:05 a.m. I squish a blue bar of goo onto my toothbrush.

Libby is in the kitchen when I walk out. Lile has taken the older boys to school and Parks is singing a song to a giant tower of foam blocks, swinging his torso from side to side. As soon as he sees me he drops his gaze, mumbles to himself, and latches onto the edge of the couch.

He's afraid of me.

Libby swats him playfully with an old, lumpy pillow and he giggles. It's probably not easy having a crazy person live in your house, but Libby acts like she's proud to have me wandering her halls in my sweatpants, thrilled to see me slowly coming back to life. I'm somehow never in her way as she flits around the room with the phone tucked between her shoulder and her chin, gossiping with her friend

Sunny from BootyBarre class, preparing snacks for the boys, and mopping up a mess that was probably never even there. I'm another hand to hold in a house full of needy, sticky fingers, but she doesn't seem to mind. She pours me juice and kisses my cheek, and when I tell her that I slept for five whole hours, she hugs me and tells me she's taking me for lunch to celebrate. My teeth are covered in moss and I haven't worn pants without a drawstring since I arrived, but still, she's proud to show me off, all disheveled and insane.

There's toast for me, two slices of wheat on a plastic Elmo plate. I sit down cautiously in front of it and stare. It's overwhelming to look at, there's too much of it, too many seeds and ten thousand spongy holes. Parks starts singing a version of "Jingle Bells."

"I love toast! I love toast! I love toasty toast."

I pick it up and insert it into my mouth. It tastes like buttered sandpaper, but two slices of toast is a victory, two slices of toast is the first mountain I climb. Parks claps for me.

The next week is mechanical. I'm just a little mouse on a wheel. There are brush bristles that graze my teeth, food that tastes like nothing on my tongue, gurgles that happen in my body, and remembering what shoe goes on what foot. I move from one non-event to the next like a lady robot trying to blend in with the real, human family she's been assigned. Feebly, I try to help around the house, but frenetic, curly-haired Libby wipes hands, cooks food, pays bills, and clips flower stems in the time it takes me to fold a single shirt. Helpless and hopeless, I resign myself to watching their happy, hectic home from the couch and wait for the joy that lives here to ping-pong off the walls and hit me in the head. It doesn't, though. Joy isn't going to just land on me: I have to find it, learn it, on my own.

The pain is real. The lightheadedness and cold sweats are real. My body nags at me for the old medicine, but each day I give it less and less, remembering what Dr. Wyatt told me. I don't go back to see her, even though I probably should. Sitting in another room waiting for a stranger in a white lab coat to tell me how to heal doesn't feel like progress anymore. What I need is to learn how to access the remedy that's already inside me, the desire to be better, the deservedness of love. I can't find that in a hospital—it just isn't a pill that they make yet.

To fill the gap between "toast" and "shower" one morning, I decide to make another list to help me navigate. I look at the pictures on the dresser and the one of my daddy beside the bed and I try to remember who I am and what it is that I like. I try to remember what *my* joy looked like before the accident and the medicine and all the shit. I squeeze my eyes shut and see Amos the mule hauling our plow across the dusty red garden, daddy in a cloud of dirt behind him. I see the big pink sun melting behind the farmhouse at the end of the day and spilling its colors all over me. I see the rocks at Camp DeSoto, where I learned what it was to be loved wholly and accepted fully. I think as hard as I can, pushing ink into the paper of a fresh section of notebook.

What did I love before pain? I ask myself.

When pain began, fear began. I haven't done anything in years that I thought might make my pain feel worse, so I've missed out on so many things that could make it feel better, make *me* feel better. It's been a long time since I've felt anything but numb. I close my eyes and just let the words come:

Sunsets
People
Dancing
Flowers
Making lists

I decide I will start with one thing, just one, every single day. Something buried deep inside me knows that the motions need to come before the emotions. If I can learn to trust that the feelings exist and move toward them, they'll come to me. It's easy to say, "Once I'm better, I'll go dancing again. Once I'm better, I'll watch the sunset again," but if you don't ever take action, find enough trust in the possibility of joy to risk the possibility of pain, you stay exactly as you are. Today, I decide to try flowers.

The afternoon is showy in its cloudlessness and so hot that the air is making that wrinkly mirage again. Peeking out the window at Libby's garden, I'm nervous about my blind date with the hydrangeas, about sitting under the live oak on the swing and waiting to feel what I used to feel. The expectation of having love for something towers over me and I worry that it's too soon to try.

The back door is heavy and the fresh air puts a shiver on my skin. It's nearly ninety-five degrees out, but the hair on my arms stands straight up. I'm in a new place: outside. I go from the dusty flats of Mars to the Amazon. I get culture shock in the backyard.

The colors spill all over each other. They compete to capture my attention, to be the loudest and brightest and boldest of the pinks or yellows. Brown birds chase each other and the neighbor's lawn mower shoots green fireworks up over the fence. There's order here, tidy edges and coiffed bushes. Azaleas are allowed to crowd the asters, and the wisteria wraps itself comfortably around a spiny-skinned rosebush. I take in all the color and light and sound.

I plop down by the camellia in the razor-blade grass and rake my fingers through the mulch until my nails are black. I wait, I beg for something beautiful, a homecoming, for the flowers to reach out and tell me they've been the answer all along, but they don't. They just sway and nod and host the butterflies. They say nothing. My head starts to ache and my throat gets narrow. I go back inside to lie down.

The next day, I try again. I open my notebook and swipe my pen through *sunsets*.

At dusk, I go to the lakes at LSU. I make Lile drop me off on his way to Jimmy John's, foregoing the stress of sandwich selection to make good on the promises I made to myself. The asphalt paths are filled with a mixture of sorority girls trying to stay a size four and old people with dogs, and the checkerboard lawn is emptier than I ever remember it being. I find a spot away from the other people and sink down onto the roots of a tree. The pain is as bad as it ever has been. I lean back into the bark and let it hold me up while a group of ducks floats slowly through the water, barely flinching as a kayak sends ripples into their sides. The sun's bottom dunks itself below the tree line. I close my eyes hard and I pray.

Make it be beautiful. Make it be beautiful. Make it be beautiful.

The edges of the sky begin to glow orange and the clouds shift from white to mauve and stretch themselves into ribbons. A pair of sprinklers spurt to life and a couple of kids perched on the edge of the water lean together into one lumpy, romantic shadow. I sit and I stare as the pinks get pinker but the sight doesn't move me—it's just science in the sky. I look over at the shadow kids again. They're making out hard with each other, all hands up the backs of legs and tongues tangling. They should probably go back to a dorm room before they make a baby in front of the mallards. It makes me feel a little something, it makes me wonder about Jack, if he misses me in Australia, if I even miss him.

Before the wondering becomes too much, the devious middle child, Rhodes, beeps the car horn, bopping up and down on Lile's lap. I walk into the smell of hot white bread and deli meat and we go home.

Joy doesn't come to me quickly the way I beg it to. Joy is something I need to cultivate. It takes time to grow, it must be nourished carefully and lovingly. I crack my pills in half, eliminating them bit by bit, one at a time, like the doctor told me to. Pain continues to rise up in me like a circus lion, and defiantly, I bully it less and less with the whip that it knows. I'm gentle with it, I'm patient. I cut down on the medicine week by week. Seven doses become six, six become five, and I try to be kind to my body as it soaks the sheets, snarls at me, and recalibrates. I follow my schedule, cling to my list, and keep trying to find little pieces of myself that had been covered over years ago by ego, pain, the story of suffering. Slowly my capacity to feel grows.

Little Lile, Rhodes, and Parks see me first. They notice I'm different even before I do, because kids are always able to peek through the veil. Something shifts, and after about two weeks of walking through the world with written directions, I'm not so scary anymore. They stop staring at me like I'm the ghost across the hall and start asking me for goldfish crackers and bursting into my room without knocking first to show off their crazy, ridiculous dance moves. Libby and Lile start to see me again too. I start washing dishes and sorting laundry and I take the car out by myself. I graduate from my plastic Elmo plate to a ceramic one.

Two weeks pass and I decide to sit by the camellias again. I wait until Libby goes to the booty class and the boys are in school, until the sun looks like it's balancing on the tops of the trees. I push the door open. My body cringes from the resistance but it's easier for me than it was the last time. I step out onto the grass barefoot. September is a hundred degrees, the leaves wilt in the middle of the day, but the ground is steady, strong, and ice-cold under my toes. It agrees to hold me up no matter what happens.

I walk toward the flowers, expecting nothing from them, but something steers me away.

Magnolia fuscata.

I say it out loud. "*Magnolia fuscata!*"

It soaks the insides of my nostrils and I swear I can see tendrils of smell floating through the air. I taste the banana smell in the back of my throat, feel the soft yellow buds on the hairs above my lip. It carries me toward the tree in the corner of the yard and I grab a glossy, honey-covered leaf between my fingers. I rub my cheek against one of the last petal clusters of the season and watch as it slowly, beautifully tumbles to the ground.

Magnolia fuscata.

The memory comes. I close my eyes and my daddy is there. We're on the farm and the smell is all around us. I see the tree covered in more flowers than it can hold, all of them the color of fresh Amish butter. It's his favorite. The red-spotted dogs are barking, bounding around him as he wipes his forehead with his handkerchief. He walks from his garden and wraps me in his arms.

"I love you more than God can count," he says to me.

I don't leave his arms for a while. I fall onto my knees and sit in my daydream, taking sips of fresh, sweet-smelling air. When I open my eyes, I can see. I can feel.

As I stand in the yard by the fragrant tree with waxy leaves, the numbness of the drugs starts to go away. The feeling of God starts to come, but it isn't the God they taught me about. She's motherly and tender and ever-loving. She's Mrs. God: poet, dear friend, and teacher. I decide that's what I'll call her for now. I recognize her from my walks in the woods at DeSoto and from the sweet-and-sour perfume of that baby I loved. I recognize her from the femininity of the Bible; the long, beautiful verses that curved and meandered; the light and song of worship. She's never left my side; she just looks different than they said she would. The white male preachers I've grown up listening to see depravity over virtue, original sin over original love, original goodness, and original purity. I don't see things that way anymore. This is my new church and all are welcome here.

The birds sing their summer carols and the tree leaves shrivel on the bottom branches that hang above me. I pluck a bud off the tree and stick it up my nose and it feels sacred, like prayer. Joy lives here; pain lives here too. As I smell the sweet blossom and heat swells up my side, I invite them both to coexist in me.

A few days later, Jack calls. He's coming back to Nashville for a weekend and I know that I need to go see him. Lile and Libby encourage me to go see him, though I'm not sure I'm ready to go away yet. Jack and I are in trouble. I can see it very clearly now. I buy a plane ticket, nervously curl the ends of my hair, and a memory comes.

I'm seven. My mom is finally making me get glasses. They're as big as windshields, with thin wire frames, and I hate them immediately when the doctor balances them on the tops of my ears. I don't like the weight of them or the look of them and I can tell they'll be a lot of work, something to push up my nose and hold in place on the monkey bars. I've decided that they're an obstacle to the important work of childhood, but I quickly learn that they're the gateway. I walk out into the parking lot afterward and I can see. I can see so much more of the world. There are bits of glitter on the parked cars and ten-color puddles underneath them. Noticing the silhouettes of birds floating miles up in the sky, I realize they're dozens of shapes, there are dozens of different bird shapes! I point and squeal and let my jaw hang low, in awe of the beauty all around me. My mom giggles and glows and the sky gets brighter and brighter. Everything is clear.

It's time to go to the airport. I look in the mirror once more, patting a ribbon of hair and rubbing my lips together. For the second time in my life, I'm starting to see again—pain, beauty, truth—and I want to share all of it with Jack.

I get back to Nashville in the early evening. The Honda is covered with leaves and sitting in its special spot by the curb. I call Lile as soon as I open the door like he made me promise to and I take myself on a tour of home.

The pretty yellow house is stuffy and strange, as though it's been left for an entire season instead of just five weeks. The kitchen is empty, the dining room table is dull and gray, and the couch is stiff. I walk into the bedroom and flop on the bed. There are little crumbs from all my snacks and my computer sits open like a dead clam. I roll onto Jack's side and trace a little heart into his pillow. I imagine our bodies lying side by side. It has been so long since we've been next to each other and so much has happened. The pills I have left rattle around in the bottom of their canister as I take them out of my purse and set them on the table where they've always lived. I can see a perfume bottle. It's been obscured by orange plastic and candy wrappers and it's so pretty, angular and made of thick, expensive glass. I fall asleep feeling guilty about it, about all the horrible things it must have seen as it stood watch there all of these years.

Jack arrives the next morning at half past nine. My body is yowling from yesterday's plane ride but I do my best to deaden the noise with hope—today isn't about me, it's about us. I hear him lug his suitcase onto the porch and catch a glimpse of the top of his head out the window. I'm anxious and nauseated and consumed by a lovely kind of fear that I remember from the first time

I climbed into the passenger seat of his car, not knowing where we would go but wanting to go anyway.

The door opens slowly and I squeal when he crosses the threshold, covered in backpacks and rumpled in all the right ways. He's exhausted from twenty-four hours in economy, flight hopping from Sydney to Nashville, and maybe just a little bloated from a touring diet of beer and Rold Gold pretzels. I am happy to see him, I think.

He throws a rigid smile at me through the jet lag and we hold each other for a long time. It's more of an awkward stuckness than an embrace. Our limbs loosen every so often, but we let the history of eight years hold us together and convince us that we are not strangers in this moment. Eventually, he steps back and the sounds of our breath bounce off the walls.

"You look really good," he says.

He doesn't really look at me, though. His eyes dart from my face to the floor to the back window. For two people who have been to opposite ends of the earth and dug into the deepest parts of themselves, we have very few stories to tell. There's a heaviness about him. I'm not sure he wants to be here, and I'm not sure that I blame him.

I giggle as he tries to untangle himself from some of the backpacks and he jumps a little, shaken by the sound of joy from me. A long pause happens and I smile at him.

"Hey, do you mind if I go to bed?" he asks. "I'm so fucking tired."

"Go!" I tell him, nodding my head and trying my best to sound airy and bright and all the things that I think he wants me to be.

He wanders away and I hear his body hit the bed like a big old tree. He sleeps through the evening.

I watch the sunrise by myself the next day while he rests in a heap on the bed. The sun is coming later and later, and though Tennessee and Louisiana are close neighbors, it's colder here in autumn than it ever is there. I think about Jack and about the heaviness. I wonder where it came from and how long it will be staying, if it's been here all along and I've been too shut inside myself to notice him buckling under the baggage I gave him. I hear him get up to take a ten-minute morning piss and all I can think about is the happiness that I owe him.

There is so much to say, but over the next two days, we become experts in silence. I keep trying to show him that I'm better, that I'm fun and easy and free. I hardly mention my pain, though it rips through my body. I prove myself by staying up late, and throwing my head back in laughter. I try to prove myself with sex, but even that is just another way to avoid talking about it all.

We mash our bodies together, kissing with stiffened jaws and touching with cold hands. All the things we don't say float over the bed above us like skywriting.

I miss you.

I'm angry.

I'm sorry.

Do you still love me?

Are you okay?

Why didn't you call?

The night before he leaves again, we pick up food from the taco shop we love and eat it on our covered back porch. There is just enough coolness in the air for us to want to sit close but we don't. Jack is slumped in a chair that hangs from the ceiling, crumbling bits of tortilla into his chicken soup and swaying back and forth. I sit facing him on a brown ottoman with not enough padding.

I look out at the fence the Amish built, their monument to my daddy. The lumber is strong and tall like he was and it still smells a little bit like the Kentucky forest it came from. He loved Jack. He delighted in him the same way he did in me, like a father is supposed to. I used to dream of him bouncing our babies on his knee, showing them how to stick watermelon seeds into the soil, whispering little secrets to them that Jack and I would never get to know. Shame and panic slink in next to me. I wonder what my daddy would think of us now.

The sun sets slowly, inch by inch by inch. Today is a sunset day for me, so I give it my full attention while Jack rocks himself. Violets and ambers and hot, hot reds wrap themselves a full 360 degrees around us and the music of rush-hour traffic plays.

I gasp at the sky.

"Look! Look up! It's beautiful!" I lean forward and touch Jack's arm but he doesn't look.

The sun gets so wide that it stretches bigger than the skyline. I point and I stand and I crane my neck so high that I have to hold the hat on my head. He still doesn't look.

I feel like I'm running out of time.

Show him something beautiful. Show him something beautiful. Show him something beautiful, I beg.

I sit back down on the ottoman and take a nervous too-big bite of corn on the cob covered in cheese. My chest is so tight the kernels barely make their way down. There are so many words caught in my throat, I can hardly swallow.

"Jack . . ." I begin hesitantly.

He brings a still-steaming spoonful of soup to his lips and immediately spits it back into its little foam cup.

"Fuck!" he sputters.

"Fuck!" he says again.

His face turns red and he sucks down half a beer.

"Fuck! Why is that so fucking hot?!"

We are not strangers to the *fuck* word; we have used it liberally, playfully, in sickness and in health. But this *fuck* is a different *fuck*. It is the satisfying, visceral *fuck* of a person who is truly angry. He abandons his soup on a table and pushes himself all the way back in his pod of a chair, and I know that this particular *fuck* has nothing to do with hot broth and everything to do with eight long years of pouring love into someone who doesn't feel it. This *fuck* is for me.

I look out at the fence again, at the pumpkin-colored sky, and then at the man who has tried and tried and might finally be done trying. I decide to be brave, and I ask him to try once more.

I stand up in front of him, because speeches are better that way, and I tell him that I'm ready. I'm ready for all of it, the vacations and the babies and a new house and all the big promises we made to each other. His eyes get wide and white.

I'm not graceful when I speak. I'm manic and excited and terrified and I go on way too long about holistic pain management and couples counseling and what I think God is and all the different ways we can start again.

"I can do it, I can live with my pain. I can carry it now, you don't have to carry it for me anymore. We can be happy. Jack, I'm so sorry. Everything is going to be different."

I hurt as I say it, badly, but I say it anyway.

He picks up his soup again and looks into it like he's reading tea leaves. Poking little pieces of cilantro and digging for shredded chicken. His face is tired. He lets me touch it, though I can tell he doesn't want me to. It feels different, older and covered with the rind of what has become a hard, hard life.

I sit down again on the ottoman, nerves tangled and burning. I brace myself for the impact of the reply, his truth telling. I ready myself to hear all the different ways I have ruined him.

But it's all too much.

He says nothing and absolutely everything at the same time.

I'm ready to meet his real, true, most damaged self, but he's not ready to introduce me yet. I understand.

Not yet, not now, be patient, his face says. So I am. It's my turn to try.

"That sounds great, babe." He sighs. "We'll set it up when the tour is done."

And he goes back to his soup.

I drive Jack to the airport the next day. We hug and kiss and say "I love you." We don't talk about my overly enthusiastic monologue on the porch with its big plans and bold proclamations. We're just nice to each other because we don't know how to be any other way. But I think, I hope, that we can learn to be more.

I go back to Louisiana after he goes. Lile and Libby don't want me to be alone yet. The morning I leave, it's cold and rainy and our pretty yellow house looks extra yellow against the charcoal of the Nashville sky.

"You're beautiful," I tell it. I make myself a promise: every time

I see something beautiful, I will speak it, declare it to myself and to the rest of the world.

The car rumbles underneath me, shaking out its chilly insides. There's a strangeness, a newness sitting with me behind the wheel. For the past seven years, I've taken this trip laid out in the back with the seat down, but today, tomorrow, and every other day from now on, the hundreds of miles between home and there are mine to conquer. The blinker clicks, the music begins, and it's time to get back to the business of healing.

That night, I settle back into Little Lile's room and stay there for another two weeks. I read and do research on the internet about chronic pain and holistic healing, I worry about my marriage constantly. One night, I come across a blog by a woman who lost both her parents, and she quotes somebody I've never heard of before named Kahlil Gibran, who I imagine is probably dead.

"The deeper that sorrow carves into your being, the more joy you can contain."

I read it twelve times in a row and make myself a promise out loud in front of no one but Mrs. God: "This is going to be my story."

I go through the motions, I cut my pills in half, I cling to my list.

16

Sex, Drums, and Lawyers

People.

It's the second item on my list. It comes after "sunsets" and before "dancing," and I just stare at the word sitting on top of its thin blue notebook line when I wake up in the morning. The six tiny letters gather weight when they stand together; they become something enormous and terrifying, a slideshow of all the people I've hurt and left broken and taken from. They come at me in a mob. Following them come the people who have left *me* broken: my daddy, who died too soon; the pastors; the Ladies in Pearls; the doctors who tried to fix me with their Easter egg–colored tablets; and sometimes, though he never means it, Jack. Shame peeks in at me. I get nervous; I pick up my little list, its edges starting to fray, and I fold it away. Most of my "people" aren't near me. I'm back in Nashville for good now. It's late September and Jack is still on tour, Katie is busy with her kids, my daddy is with Mrs. God. I need to find new people for myself before the isolation, the medication, the loss of hope begin again.

I meet Allie at the end of the month. She's a musician and lives just down the street from us in a tiny '70s duplex with windows shaped like diamonds. It sits across the street from an identical '70s duplex with a yard full of barking Rottweilers that make me jump when I walk by. My old Bible study friend Katherine introduces us; they met at camp or school or church. Something like that.

"You know, Allie just needs to find her people," Katherine muses on the phone.

I *do* know. I need to find my people too. I used to find my people in church, but I haven't been in ages, and I'm not sure I'll ever go back. I'm tired of the transaction: expectation and betrayal, reward and entitlement, the rising costs of salvation. Faith is different for me: my God gives graciously, forgives freely, and teaches endlessly. She asks for nothing in return but love. Now, though, I'm not sure where to find my people, so when Katherine calls, I decide to find fellowship with someone called Allie who is also looking.

One night, Katherine and I walk down the bright white sidewalks to Allie's house with a cheese pizza. RUF taught me that it's easier to find fellowship with food. We all eat together sitting on cinder blocks underneath the rusty, corrugated carport that's too short to house her big white van and stands in as a patio instead. I like Allie right away, which is a relief. She's sweet and funny and deep and asks the most thoughtful questions. She has a three-year-old son named Gabriel. Her eyes get wide and peaceful when she talks about him, going on about how he doesn't like sleeping in his own bed or broccoli, how he's a billion watts of brightness and energy and perfection, how she can't wait for me to meet him. I listen and nod and think about what it must be like to raise a child alone in a big city, to travel through a new world and be expected to guide someone else. I get my own motherly feeling, a call to protect her and help her, whatever that looks like. I don't want her to have to be alone. Conveniently, I don't want to be alone either.

Deep into autumn, I visit Allie and Gabriel nearly every day. We play in the dirt and count freckles, first the ones on his nose, then the ones on his mom's. In the evenings, we meet across from the big barking dogs and walk along the wide white sidewalks until supper. Gabriel darts ahead and pauses to blow big soapy bubbles out of his plastic wand while Ellie waddles behind us. I watch them together, see him tuck his hand into hers, hear the song she sings to him about waking up in the morning, and motherhood cries out to me. We eat lots of takeout dinners together on the cinder blocks, and when we sit there talking all bundled up, I feel like I'm perched on the worship rocks at DeSoto again. I tell her my everything, about Jack and being on drugs and getting off drugs and wanting a family. She tells me her everything, too, about being in love, getting pregnant and divorced, and after all of it, still wanting love more than anything else in the world. Wordlessly, we make an agreement to be there for each other. She's the first person I meet since losing myself to pain who trusts in me enough to lean on me.

I babysit Gabriel for her as often as I can. After a long night playing at the bar where they serve two-dollar cans of PBR, she comes home exhausted. The guitar case slams against the doorjamb when she drags it inside; her top lip is covered with snot from her runny nose. She tries to smile big at me, but I know she's pretending. I know what it is to pretend that way. We look in at her son, asleep in a room as bright as a tanning bed, and God says something through her.

"Thank you for taking such good care of us."

I hold her for a long time, lovingly, the way my daddy held me. The words are such a gift. I've been working hard, cutting back on the medicine bit by bit, soothing myself through the night sweats and dizzy spells and surges of pain. Every pill I've snapped in half and swallowed down has held fear and hope inside, and today it feels like hope is bigger. Just a month ago, I couldn't even take care of myself.

Helping Allie becomes a new kind of medicine, though it can never really heal me. Attempting to rescue someone else from their pain just distracts me from my own. I show up for her daily with open arms, ready to be useful but really, ready to *feel* useful. Looking outside myself to be the answer to somebody else's problems is easier than looking inside to find the answers to my own. I'm loyal, steadfast, and kind. Tentatively but joyfully, I let her believe in me. I begin to believe in myself.

Jack's on the road when I tell him about Allie, about the babysitting, about the long, winding walks, about the conversations that go on too late. Our phone calls are short and flat, debriefings.

"That's great, babe," he mutters through the phone. I'm not sure where he is, but he sounds further away than he's ever been before.

We isolate when we're suffering, and Jack is still suffering. He hides it differently than I do, on a tour bus outside Denver instead of in a bed, but it's hiding all the same. I want him to see that I'm ready, that I can show up for him, but the harder I try to reveal myself, the less he wants to look.

"I made a new friend!"

He sighs, like all he can see is a recluse.

"I walked two miles today!"

He rushes off the phone, like all he can see is a cripple.

"My doctor says I'm the poster child for healing!"

He says he needs to say goodbye and I feel like he can't even see me.

"I love you!"

It's like all he can hear is *I need you.*

"We'll talk again soon," he says, while beer bottles clink in the background and people say muffled cusswords. There's laughter and he laughs, too, at a joke he'll never explain to me. It used to be "tomorrow," but now it's just "soon."

I keep working on me so that eventually, he'll want to work on us. I see a holistic pain doctor who gives me vitamins and teaches me stretches and cheers me on with clinical enthusiasm. I take yoga classes and Pilates classes and get therapeutic massages to try to make my body a more peaceful place to live. I read books about how to heal chronic pain and books about how to heal my relationships, which remind me how little control I have over them. I can only try to heal myself. I try my best, balancing the pain inside me, the relentless burn, with the beauty that exists outside it. It's the only salve that seems to work.

Nashville is a gray slab covered in wet leaves and pumpkin guts when Jack finally comes home. I hope that through the bad weather and empty, *Sleepy Hollow* streets, he'll be able to find something beautiful here, that maybe I could be the something beautiful. I've been weaning myself off the drugs alone for more than three months now and I know I'm doing a good job. The anxiety is real, the new-old pain is real, but I survive them. I don't let them steer me anymore. I take control of our life too. I pay bills, buy fresh produce, and get the oil changed in the cars, making painstaking preparations for the unveiling of me.

I clean the house from top to bottom the day he gets in. It's a strange museum tour, traveling slow down the hall, wiping down artifacts of our life together that I can hardly remember. I dust the spot on the bedside table where the orange pill canisters used to live; I pull up the cover on the red rolltop desk and find a grainy picture of my daddy when he was a little boy, pants pulled up high, hair parted on the side and slicked down. I stare into the lumpy glass of the big, lagoon-colored jars on the kitchen counter that have been waiting years for the sugar, flour, and coffee beans they were made to hold. I pick one up and smile at my funny, Smurf-ish reflection, just one empty vessel looking into another. Feeling peaceful and flooded with gratitude, I untack the garbage bags from the window as gently and intentionally as Jack placed them there. I wave to God as she blows through the buck-naked branches of the dogwood trees.

Landed.

He texts at 4:30 p.m. and the sun's already setting. I put on new clothes that don't smell like Scrubbing Bubbles and wait for him on the porch, goose bumps rising on my arms when I open the door. It's cold, I'm nervous, and I hope he likes the tower of decorative gourds I stacked up under the mailbox. Small teardrop-shaped leaves tumble down in corkscrews to blanket the sidewalk in yellow and I say a prayer with my hands tucked under my armpits. *Let it be enough, let me be enough.*

The headlights approach. It's not his car, but somehow, I know he's inside. The glow gets closer and brighter and I just wait for what's happening to happen. The passenger-side door opens, he climbs out all scruffy and perfect, and the car drives away.

"Hey."

A too-big breath of air pushes down my throat and makes an ache in my chest.

"Hey." I can hardly get it out.

I'm not sure what I want him to see, a new person he can love, the old person he used to love, hopefulness, healing, something different from what he left behind. I pull him into my arms before he can decide what I am to him.

I'm not numb anymore.

I don't say it. I want to, but I don't. It can't be about me anymore, not the way it has been. We stand there for a minute in the wetness while the cars whiz by. I soak up the weight and the warmth of him and let his long, wordless exhale tickle my earlobe. It takes a minute, but he curls his big long arms around me and holds on to me. *He's still holding on to me.*

The next few days are full of trying. We go on dates and stay up too late and visit our therapist, Jane, in the suburbs. She tries to help us navigate all the different ways we've hurt each other. Jack says he's tired and angry and confused by me, that I'm a totally different person now. Quietly, I let it crush me because I thought that's exactly what he wanted. I forgive him for everything I possibly can in that room because I want him to forgive me, too, I want to force the transaction, settle the settlement and move on, but he isn't ready for total restitution.

We want to make it work, but we don't know how to.

"I love you."

"I love you too."

It's the only thing we can agree on, but neither of us really knows what it means anymore. Jane just stares at us, nodding and making notes. She doesn't know what it means either.

We're lying on top of the covers of our big sleigh bed when he says it, matter-of-factly.

"I'm going back out."

It's only been a week, but Jack wants to leave again.

The beginnings of rain start in. I close my eyes, swallow hard, and listen.

"They're counting on me."

He rubs my arm and we both look up, searching for words on the ceiling.

But I'm counting on you. Again, I just think it, but he pops his head up from the pillow like he knows.

The raindrops keep coming and we stay silent, listening to the water smack against the windows in intervals, watching it slide down to the ledge in pretty rivers. I wonder if he's noticed that I took the trash bags down. I wonder if it means anything to him. The weather gets louder and time to speak shrinks away. I feel my pulse rise up to my temples. We need more time.

"Please don't go. You'll miss Thanksgiving."

I've never asked him to stay before. It surprises both of us.

"We need this." It crackles out of me, I'm a pitchy sixth-grade boy. "I'm almost off all the pills. I've never asked you to stay before. The kids will be there. It'll be our first—"

"Babe, I can't. I'm sorry."

I put my head on his chest and let a tear roll across the bridge of my nose and down onto his T-shirt. It's been a long time since I've let him come close enough to hurt me. I let another one drop and another. His arm rises and he rolls my body into his. The wanting-to-love-me seeps out of him, but so does the impossibility. He's going away again. I can't make him stay. I can't make him do anything.

He tries a fix of his own.

"Hey, let's get out of town. Just for a few days."

Allie and Gabriel stay at our house to dog-sit for the weekend while we drive five hours to Asheville, North Carolina, a village of delicious restaurants in the Blue Ridge Mountains. We wander around the antique shops and eat tapas and have sex that feels better than I remember sex feeling before. We try to remember the picture of life that we drew when he first put his great-grandmother's ring on my finger and add onto it in frantic scribbles: we could adopt a baby, we could go on more vacations, get a bigger house, get a bigger dog, the ideas go on and on. I say yes to all of them, and eventually, as we dream at each other across restaurant tables, the scribbles start to look something like a picture, a future, the answer.

I call Allie from the hotel to check in and tell her about all the big plans. My heart is beating in the back of my throat and I'm talking too fast.

"That's awesome, Ruthie," she says.

I can hear Gabriel overfilling Ellie's bowl in the background; kibble tumbles from the bag out onto the floor. Giggles tumble out of Gabriel.

"Shit!" Allie whisper-shouts.

She remembers something. "Hey, I'm so sorry but I broke one of those blue jar things in the kitchen last night."

For a reason I can't name, I see the jar in big blue chunks in my mind and there's grief. I shove it away.

"It's totally fine. No big deal," I promise, and we say goodbye.

I cry about it while Jack showers. It's a silly and embarrassing, bulldozing sadness. I wipe my eyes with a corner of pillow and try not to sniff too hard, but Jack notices. I tell him about the jar and make my tears into a joke about hormones. He smiles, looks at me like I'm crazy, and kisses my head.

"It's just an empty jar. There wasn't even anything in it."

"I know." I smile and I picture it. Clear and blue, it stood ready for years to be filled up. Now it's too late.

When we get home, we start over immediately and furiously before doubt has the slightest chance to creep in. The first thing we do is sell the pretty yellow house. The neighborhood has gone from hovel to hot spot over the past eight years and with the sale, there'll be more than enough money for us to find a new place for our new beginning, its babies and dinner parties, for its big, tall Christmas tree.

Jack has to go back out on the road, but this time I feel like he might miss me. I drop him off at the airport, kiss him, and promise that I'll take care of everything, the house stuff, the bank stuff, the decorating, and that's exactly what I do. I beam as I sell the pretty yellow house and the furniture that we don't need, as I diligently hire a cleaning company, pick up rolls of packing tape, and throw a yard sale. Best of all, on one of December's darkest, most blustery afternoons, I peel off my very last fentanyl patch, which has taken four months for me to wean myself from. Allie and Gabriel keep me company while Jack is gone. They help me wrap the bits of our life we want to take with us in soft strands of newspaper and we place them into sandy-brown boxes. It doesn't cross my mind that some of the boxes will never be unpacked.

Just in time for New Year's Eve, Jack and I move into a big blue "beginning again" house. All our beautiful things come with us: the remaining blue jars (I fill them with cookies and cereal bars right away), the red rolltop desk, and our old sleigh bed. The ugliness stays behind: not a single orange canister of pills or medical bill is allowed through the door. We slow-dance between the boxes, singing the New Year's song they sing at the end of *It's a Wonderful Life* and looking around at our new space. Flat white paint covers the walls, the fridge is wrapped in plastic, and the lawn is still green even though it's winter. The rest of the street is a jealous patch of stringy brown stalks and mud. Jack likes the ceilings the best. They're so high, we could have church in the living room. I like the upstairs study—it'll be a bedroom for our oldest.

Over the next two weeks, I try to make our new space look like "us," even though we're still trying to figure out what "us" looks like. There's a big fiddle-leaf fig plant and clearance wallpaper from Anthropologie, a comfortable chair and flat-screen television. I gather enough linens and living room furniture to last us a lifetime, but our life together only goes on for another month.

Jack and Allie are making a record together. He's always wanted to produce something, and when I introduced them back in November, I hoped that they would work together. Gabriel stays with me while they're in the studio. We play trains on the shockingly new floors and eat Teddy Grahams for dinner because I'm still not very good at cooking. My body aches more and more these days, but I can't resist lifting him up, spinning him around, and dreaming of my own child. As I watch his long, feathery lashes come together and his wiry boy body settle into sleep, I find solace and purpose and peace. I know that I'm ready to be a mom. On these late nights of trains and bear-shaped cookies, Gabriel and I grow close. So do Allie and Jack.

At first, I hardly detect it. I watch Jack's entire body lift off the ground when she knocks at our front door, I watch him tell Gabriel jokes and carry him on his shoulders, I watch his face grow softer when he says her name. It's so unimaginable, I think the new joy in him must be for me and I welcome it. Allie's china-doll cheeks grow pink when he looks at her; she starts to dress up for recording sessions and put lipstick on. I watch all of it happen, but I never believe in a world where Jack isn't my devoted, patient husband and Allie isn't my closest friend, where I'm not the link that joins them together.

In February, Katherine and I go to watch Allie play a show at 3rd and Lindsley, the same old club near the interstate where Jack and I began our life together. For the second time I see him illuminated in that dank little room, resurrected from his heaviness. He watches her on the stage like she's levitating; he laughs and drinks and comes to life. I feel happy for him, for us, and I wonder if we need to get out more often.

"I don't like this," Katherine says, her denim-colored eyes getting small and angry, darting from Allie, drenched in perfect golden light, to Jack, drenched in Allie, to me. Still, I don't believe it. He runs over to the stage after the show and helps her lift her guitar from her shoulder; they stare at each other and whisper. I don't know what they're saying, but their mouths are open wide in laughter. I laugh along with them like I'm a part of it all.

"Do you guys want to come out with us?" Jack's eyes are so molten chocolate they're giving off heat. He stares at Katherine and me, waiting for an answer. He's so consumed that he doesn't even realize he's inviting his wife to go out with him and another woman. I'm so unthreatened that I hardly notice either and don't think twice about heading home so they can enjoy the rest of the night together. Katherine does, though.

"I don't like this," she says one more time as their shadows grow closer in the doorway behind us. I begin to feel nervous, not because I think Jack would be unfaithful, he never would be, Allie wouldn't either, there are lines neither one of them would cross, but because the look of happiness in both of them seems so pure. Jack and I haven't been that way in a long time. That night, Jack comes home late and sleeps in the guest room.

About a week passes. Jack and I sit facing each other in the big blue house we bought so that we could begin again, and we end there, badly, painfully, in tears.

"I know you want to be a mom more than anything in the world. I'm going to be a dad one day, I'm going to be an amazing dad."

It comes out of nowhere and he can't even look me in the eye. Every single syllable reverberates off the ceilings he loves and makes a hard landing under my ribs. The admission feels so deliberate, an expertly engineered final straw. I don't try to stop myself from crying. He doesn't need to continue, but he does.

"You want a child more than you want me," he continues. "And I'll never do it. Not with you."

There is a silence, a quiet, empty nothingness, where neither one of us can speak or move. Our breaths drift into each other and in our very last moments together, I'm broken wide open. The pain is real and visceral, it has a pulse of its own. I listen to him as he dismantles our life beside the new fiddle-leaf fig plant, but his words don't make any sense. I thought he wanted all of it as much as I did. All I ever wanted was to be able to give it to him. My voice shakes for just a second and then I erupt. He's wrong, he's being ridiculous, he's cruel, he's an asshole. Nothing I say can touch him.

I get up from the couch and I leave. There isn't enough air in the house we bought so that we could breathe again. I spend the night at Katherine's, crying into her hair.

It's evening the next day when I return home, and before I go in, I stand out in the crunchy, frost-covered yard and stare at the sky. It's a "sunset" day and the most beautiful tangerine blob is melting over the cold city; it all goes from orange to purple to blue. I'm in shambles, sharing the lawn with our perfect new home and looking up at it with longing because even six feet away it feels so out of reach.

Jack isn't waiting for me when I open the door. I don't know where he is or if he's ever coming back. Allie stops returning my calls. I feel like I lose them both in the same instant. It hurts, but what hurts most is that the end of us isn't about Jack and Allie, it's about Jack and me. We haven't been in love in a long time. It would be easier if there were a wild affair, if this were about the power of their love, but it's about the tiredness of ours. I *feel* tired.

The sounds my sneakers make on the floor float through the dead air and reverberate on the wall. I'm alone. I think of my list and I cling to it once again.

17

A Come-to-Justin Meeting

The forest in South Louisiana is a giant stick monster that crawls up from the swamp. There are creeping plants and brambles and long-limbed trees that can never quite pull themselves from the muck, so they grow sideways instead. There are snakes that can swim and gators and beautiful brown deer, birds that cackle at you when you walk and thick, buzzing gnat clouds that smack you in the eye. Some people are scared of the forest, but it was my playground; I could explore it for hours with just my juice box, a dog or two, and a walking stick, climbing, digging, and swinging from tree to tree.

The vines are everywhere. They hang down in long, skinny car-wash curtains, leathery and strong. I'd stand on a stump, beat my xylophone ribs like Tarzan, grab ahold, and just soar, howling back to the jungle that howled to me, called me out from the house and reminded me that I could be wild and free. Flying forward was euphoric; everything blurred into a brown, manic swirl of leaves and limbs and noises. Flying the other way was terrifying. The motion slowed, the sweat on my hands became a slick grease, the sickness from taking flight settled in my stomach. Then, blindly, faster and faster and faster, I'd go backward.

When Jack leaves, everything that's good, moving ever forward, begins to slow. A sickness comes, and I fall back, blindly, faster and faster and faster. I land in bed, the most comfortable and dangerous place in the world.

I wake up alone in the big blue house. My lips are dry as tree bark and there's brown sludge on my face. Long muddy streaks stretch across the perfect white pillow that Jack abandoned one week ago; it looks like dried blood. I touch my face, search my mouth for the nickel-y taste of a bitten cheek. Instead, I find a sweetness in the back of my mouth that jolts me. The night comes back to me: sobbing, sleeplessness, loneliness, the heating pad to help with my back and to stand in for the warm body that went away. Chocolate. A shard of Skinny Cow wrapper peeks out from the long gaps of my left hand; a tiny ball of nougat is curled up in my palm. Just because I'm not on fentanyl doesn't mean I don't medicate.

There are things I love in the world, but today I don't choose them. Yesterday I didn't choose them. Jack is gone and the future is an empty place now. The little list that held my hand is sitting under a mug next to a stack of mail that belongs to the man who may not come back. It stays there because it's easier to anesthetize myself with Cosmic Brownies from the gas station, extra pillows, and season seven of *The Millionaire Matchmaker* than it is to put on my pants and open the door.

My phone blinks at me. Obediently, I roll to it and let rainbow sprinkles clatter onto the floor from inside my T-shirt.

8:00 a.m. Get out of bed.

I obey, but only because all the snacks have melted. Blood flies dizzily up to my brain and the pain says good morning the way it always does, rushing up my side in a big hot blaze. I walk to the shower where Jack and I joked we would make a baby and I feel myself swinging backward, body scared and stiff, through the brown, swirling forest, faster and faster and faster.

The most terrifying thing about Jack being gone and Allie being gone is that I've lost my "people," the other heartbeats that bump alongside my own and confirm to me that I'm not alone sixty-five times per minute. I see my reflection best when it bounces off the ones I love, I always have, and without them, I don't really know who I am. Amber comes over in the evening to watch an episode of *The Bachelor* with me. She's a new friend. She lives with my massage therapist, who works from home, and though I hardly know her from anything other than making small talk in the waiting room/living room, I invite her over because she mentions that she's going through a breakup too.

Amber is familiar, a tiny blond hummingbird with glowy ice-blue eyes and a heart that's too big for her body, just like Tim's wife, Laura. She plops down next to me on the couch, and together, we watch in inexplicable awe as a nervous boy from Texas ogles girls in slinky dresses pulling their slinky bodies out of limousines. Either everything we're watching is fake or all a person needs to find love is an application and an adult-size quinceañera dress. We eat four cupcakes between us and roll our eyes while we think about it.

A commercial for Cymbalta comes on. A happy, pain-free woman sits with her dalmatian, stares at the sky, and thinks about how wonderful life has been since the little pills showed up. I don't really want to talk, but it comes out of me anyway.

"Jack's gone."

The Texas boy is back on the screen now. He talks with a schoolteacher with no eyebrows left, then a bartender. He pulls at his bow tie and drinks a sweaty drink as a line of sequins and boobs forms behind him.

"I know. I'm so sorry," Amber says.

She tilts her beautiful, familiar face and looks me in the eyes. She reminds me so much of Laura, I forget that she's not and ask her a hundred questions she can't answer.

"Should I get a lawyer?"

"Can I get a job?"

"Am I ever going to be a mother?"

"Is it really over?"

The boy from Texas blushes in front of a fountain and I fall to pieces. She holds on tighter and I let her sister me awhile.

"Ruthie, my husband left me too. He had an affair."

I think about Allie and Jack and wonder if they're together right now, if they're curled up on a couch somewhere, her head resting in the spot on his shoulder that mine used to. The picture of it makes my stomach twist and shrink. In a measured, calm, and loving tone, Amber continues.

"It was terrible for both of us. Nobody wants a marriage to end. Nobody wants to hurt the person they swore to God they would protect. It wasn't what either of us imagined. We loved each other, just like you and Jack."

She talks about her ex with grace and care; there's no anger, no judgment, only empathy. Her glacier eyes melt a little bit and her soothing sisterly voice gets quieter. She's sad but she's gracious, she's hurt but she's healing. She doesn't make a monster of him or a saint of herself.

The Texas boy sends a gaggle of long-necked women back to their Midwest marketing jobs and they cry all over their sequins.

If Jack and I really do split up, I want to see our ending just like Amber saw hers. I don't want to be bitter. To be angry at somebody who has loved the most faded version of you, held you as you buried your father, changed your dressings so that your wounds are allowed to become scars, somebody who sat quietly on their own mountain of hurt until they knew you were able to climb down from yours, feels cheap and empty, a betrayal of its own. Whatever happens, I want it to happen with love.

They play the clips from next week. A girl with gigantic hair gets a kiss and the cameras try to make chemistry where it doesn't exist. Out of bravery or desperation, I ask Amber a question I've never asked anyone before.

"Amber, what if this is it? What am I going to do with my life?"

She sits up straight, leans in, and speaks the words straight into me.

"You'll live it." She nods, reminding herself too. "You'll do what you love. You'll do what makes you happy."

Happy. I think about it for a second.

"The only thing that makes me happy right now is Justin Timberlake."

She laughs and claps her hands, but I'm dead serious.

In hardship, some people turn to Jesus, but I turn to Justin. He's a better dancer.

It's the second week of March. Justin Timberlake is releasing a new record and he's going to be on *Jimmy Fallon* every single night for a whole week. It's a Christmas miracle. It's the opportunity, it's Mrs. God throwing a bucket of ice water over my head.

My list has grown old and velvety under the mug, but as soon as I hear about Timberweek, I revive it. I write JUSTIN in letters that are twice as big as they need to be. I'm mortified that it took me so long to give him his spot there.

It begins the evening of March 13 in my living room. Justin is on TV wearing a T-shirt, jeans, and a leather jacket; I'm on the couch wearing my big brown slippers, an old T-shirt of Jack's, and a pair of old cotton panties from college. There are purplish-blue lights, leather, and brass, a mass of beautiful people crammed into a too-tiny camera frame. I turn the volume up as loud as it goes and the sky-high ceilings of our big blue house fill up with soul. I'm finally having church here the way I wanted to.

The band and the dancers move together in their street clothes and the guitar moans along with them in long, echoey notes. Their reflections bounce off the bells of the trumpets and the saxophones, and they all cut up under the colored heat of the lights.

I know this scene. I sit straight up.

I feel like I'm looking in on a dance at West Feliciana with Pam and Miguel and Jamise. Justin's crew moves like mine, not in sync, but in solidarity. They make space for each other as he sings to them and I remember showing off in our little circle. Even though I looked ridiculous, they loved me more and more every time my skinny butt hit the gym floor.

Justin hits the highest note and I miss being sixteen so much it could crack me open.

"Yes. Fuck. Yes." There's nobody here to tell but it needs to be said. I've never heard a man make that sound before. He's a sexy jungle bird.

I close my eyes and I swim in his voice, his joy, his party.

Suddenly, I feel it. My chin starts bopping. The drummer is way back in the shot, and he's bopping too. I think about Jack, about moving my body to his music on the side stage back in Austin, nerves shot, like the buzzing copper innards of electrical wire. I danced for him, desperately, with everything, just wanting him to see me and to remind him I was still there under the drug haze and the days spent in bed. He never did see, but of course he didn't. I never saw myself either.

The drummer on TV comes down on the cymbal and I put my hands up.

The song stops being a thing that happens outside my body; it becomes my breath and my blood. I pry myself up. The comfort of the couch is an adhesive, but Justin won't let me be stuck to something right now. Like a holy miracle on a big, carpeted church stage, I'm dancing, for the first time in years.

Percussion leads me ecstatically around the room and makes my feet light. I grind and make cursive letters with my butt while Ellie stands up on the couch and flicks her pom-pom tail. I smile big at her, I cry, and I hoot and sing until my lungs ache more than my back does. Every movement is a fight, but what a fucking fight! What a blissful rebellion!

The end comes. Way too soon. Horns begin to exhale, lights scramble back and forth. I join Justin for one last, euphoric scream, and I see her. I catch a wobbly glimpse of myself in the window, made by nighttime into a wall of dark mirrors.

There she is.

Joyful, silly, soulful. Radically sacred. Pajamas and sweat and freedom. There *I* am.

Springtime is filled with silence from Jack and loudness from the rest of the world. He's everywhere in the big blue house. His clothes hang next to mine in our closet, and three pairs of big, boat-shaped tennis shoes huddle together by the front door, but I rarely hear from him. I call him; he doesn't answer. I text; I'm not even sure he reads the messages. I don't know if this is what it looks like when a marriage is over or if there's some way we can begin again *again*. When the quiet gets too quiet, when the pain keeps me awake at night, and when I hunger for Jack's body next to mine, I call on the new and old heartbeats—Amber's, Katherine's, and, of course, Justin's—they stand beside me in song. We all gather together in the evenings for dancing and grieving and whiskey drinks that get hot in our throats. We fill up the empty spaces of the big blue house and I keep fighting to catch more glimpses of myself. By April, I feel a hundred years older than I did in March. Chronic pain, by definition, doesn't really get better, but I try to live with it as best I can. I take care of my body by exercising it, dragging it along the sidewalks under the cherry trees, feeding it whatever it wants. I surround it with beauty, the single most effective medication I've tried. I find it in the daylilies opening up wide to receive the sun; in backyard dance parties; in dark, syrupy rum drinks and the feeling of fellowship. I find it hiking at Burgess Falls, where the rocks are electric green with moss and water sings to me louder than my broken nerves and broken heart can scream. Pain is big, but beauty is bigger. I make beauty my mission.

Looking for love on the outside to fill the pit on the inside, I start an Instagram account. I document everything that feels beautiful to me, from the biggest adventure to the smallest decorating project. My following grows and I use social media as a place I can go to lose myself and find myself all at once. The woman I am there is strong and pretty. Her life is fabulous. She has enough friends. Every "like" feels like love; every follower feels like an admirer. I post twice a day, three times a day, sometimes more. It's a new addiction that's impossibly easy to feed.

18

The Yes Thing

There's a Walmart nearby that thinks it's a grocery store. They sell two different types of lettuce and the cashiers wear green smocks. Even without the stretchy pants and plastic baby pools and polyester flowers, you still know exactly where you are. Sad gray lights are in cages, sad gray produce gets misted too much and hunches over, and people hunch over, too, preoccupied, irritated, wanting to get in and out without being seen. I started shopping there after Jack left, shuffling around in my sweatpants and looking lost like the rest, using it as a refuge when I didn't want to feel so alone in the hardness of life.

The store is busy today. People are hurling packages of cheap pink hot dogs and jugs of neon Faygo soda into their carts. It's May and everybody is grilling out: salt and smoke waft up and down the streets from 4 p.m. to midnight, and ketchup-stained paper plates peek out from too-full garbage cans. I love the early celebrations of summer, but I just buy a keg of laundry detergent, some peanut butter M&M's, and a plastic container of berries. Jack is still gone and still silent, so I don't need much to get by.

Randi at checkout wears her glasses on a long string of beads and smiles at me the way we all smile at each other in Walmart when I roll my almost-empty cart up to her.

It'll get better, right? I wonder, smiling big.

She gives me a tired but earnest grin in return as she bleeps and bloops my things over the scanner.

The people are getting restless behind me. They have places to go and hot dogs to grill, but I just have Randi. I don't rush her.

I hand her my card and she swipes it lazily through the reader. It doesn't work.

"Let's try it again, honey," she grumbles, coughing cigarette smell at me.

She swipes again. It still doesn't work. Her saggy bloodhound eyes fill with knowingness. The line becomes palpably furious; it shifts and sighs behind me while the blood surges up into my sinuses.

Randi smiles at me regretfully, a stiff line of lips and wrinkles.

"It's okay, sugar. Why don't you come back and see me later?"

I nod. It takes me a minute to understand, but Randi breaks it to me gently with her dog eyes.

He's not coming back. It's over.

We don't have any money and I don't know why. Maybe Jack's having a slow month? Maybe he hasn't been working at all? We didn't talk much about the finances or the mortgage or the cost of living. We never talked about the fact that I didn't work and my disability check barely covered the water bill. It felt impolite to talk about money, even after almost a decade, but now, I don't have any and the man who's been supporting me rarely returns my calls. That doesn't feel very polite either.

I know I should put my groceries away, but I abandon them next to some pale ears of corn and shuffle fast to the car. I sit crying behind the wheel and wonder how it is that a game of house turns into a game of Battleship.

Laura calls. I'm still in the parking lot, hysterical and broke, and I tell her everything she needs to know in a single word.

"Over."

She shushes me and tells me she loves me, comforting me the way only moms know how to. I can hear the farmhouse creak through the phone as the instincts left over from five babies rock her back and forth.

"You're not alone in this, Ru. We're with you all the way."

Tim comes on. He's stoic and understanding and nonjudgmental, wildly himself. He wires me two thousand dollars. I'm so embarrassed I can hardly stand to thank him for it.

I go back home to the big blue house knowing that we'll probably have to sell it, carve up what it's worth in a conference room with lawyers and a big table. I stuff my face into the pillow that used to be Jack's and wonder how it all happened, how the man who held me up and walked me around the block in a neck brace can't find enough love in him to talk to me on the phone except on the rarest occasion.

That afternoon, I post a picture of our old pretty yellow house on Instagram and think about him. I let the memories we made there gnaw at me for a minute: collecting antiques, wallpapering, planning the nursery, scribbling away at a future that would end up in the trash shortly before Valentine's Day 2013. I wonder what the hell I'm going to do now.

Over the next few days, I want to be angry, I want to sit and stew and hurt, but reality comes at me, and I can't. I either need to find a job or move back to St. Francisville to take up grieving lost love full-time with my mom. I look on Craigslist and Monster.com; I check the neighborhood newspaper and the crumbling bulletin board at the YMCA where people pin their posters about getting rich quick and the hard-core toddler swimming lessons where they just toss them in the water and hope for the best. There are plenty of jobs out there but I haven't worked in years and I don't even feel qualified to scoop ice cream or groom a dog. I don't know what to do, so I send Mrs. God a prayer about it. She replies with an email three days later.

I'm on the set of a Christmas photo shoot. It's summertime and it's so hot that the tinsel is wilting. Silver flecks are everywhere, in our hair, in our fingernails, in the cracks of our asses. We dance around our kitschy white tree singing Bing Crosby and wrapping ourselves in fat, fruit punch–colored twinkle lights. A singer named Brandon is releasing a holiday record, and last week, the photographer shooting his record cover asked me if I'd work as a stylist. It took me two terrified, unprepared, aching days to reply but I said yes. I don't have the luxury of no—it isn't an option when you don't know how you're going to pay your bills. You can't worry about what your body can handle and what it can't. You just have to move forward.

Brandon walks out from the kitchen wearing felt antlers and a patchwork sweater-vest covered in wool sugar cookies. We both start laughing.

"Yes" brought me here. It doesn't just open the doors, it bull-dozes them.

I become a stylist. I'm not exactly sure how it happens, but it feels almost like it happens without my knowledge. People find pictures of the big blue house on Instagram and the pretty yellow house on *Design*Sponge*. They like the Taylor Swift album cover that was shot at my house and the table settings I design for friends' dinner parties. All at once, I start to get messages asking about my rates and availability and I'm so surprised that I don't even know what to say. Amber does, though.

"Ruthie, does styling make you happy?"

I nod and blink at her.

"Does designing make you happy?"

I nod again.

"Then what are you waiting for? Say *yes!*"

So I do. And I keep saying it.

I'm thirty-three years old. I never knew I was creative, that I had a skill, let alone a talent. The feelings of shame and doubt and ineptitude were so big for so long that I thought all I could do was take from people. I never thought I could serve them. The story of worthlessness, of shame, is woven tightly into me, but just because you know a story by heart doesn't mean it's true.

I spend July visiting flower farms, searching for the perfect fragrant bundle of lavender, hosting events for magazines and brands I love, and learning how to haggle with the vendors at the Nashville Flea Market. I decorate and I curate and I network. At first, I don't make much money, if any. Sometimes I even end up spending a little of my own just to get a job done right. What I do get is pride, confidence, and the joy of not just seeing beauty, but creating it. I get the most wonderful friends, too, a beautiful, hilarious, ever-expanding soul family.

The work is hard on my body, standing over dinner tables adjusting sprigs of rosemary, staying on my feet for nine hours, pulling outfits and lugging furniture. It's hard on my heart too. In every kid's room I decorate, I remember the one I planned for our baby with the red rolltop desk, the old map of Louisiana, and my daddy's handkerchief tied to the mobile. In every full family home, I feel the emptiness of my own and picture Jack playing trains with Gabriel at Allie's. He's moved on but he hasn't sent divorce papers; he's left me but hasn't bothered to pick up his things. It's like he's just forgotten. For me, the feeling is worse, I think, than being left and at least remembered.

Tim is so excited to see me doing something other than eating Twinkies in bed that he helps me pay for a website that I don't really know how to use at first. I meet the quiet, petite graphic designer at a coffee shop. She drinks a giant cup of green tea and uses a pencil to hold her hair out of her eyes. We pick out a template together and she explains how I'll upload photos and blogs in computery words that I've heard before but don't understand. I nod furiously at her, more out of excitement than comprehension.

When she asks me what I want to call it, I hesitate. The pause isn't long but it's thoughtful. My mind returns to my most joyful place, singing and dancing on the porch with my mom in the kitchen and my daddy in the garden, both just within my view.

"Ruthie Lindsey Design."

Jack isn't coming back, I just know it. But Ruthie Lindsey is.

She smiles and asks me to spell it out for her letter by letter. I'm sad but certain.

I order a giant stack of business cards when people start asking for them, and I have RUTHIE LINDSEY DESIGN embossed on those too. The letters are raised high as they can be into thick ivory cardstock and they're filled with rich, leathery ink. The UPS man thunks them down on the porch, and when I gently slide the first one out and hold it in my hand, it feels more like a birth announcement. A new person is here. I run my fingertips over the words and start to cry.

"Ruthie Lindsey."

My mom's excited too. I'm not sure she understands exactly what I do, but she's so proud that she shows off my website to all her friends and they all join Instagram to follow me. She's doing better, just like I am. We both still need to cling to our lists some days, but miraculously, we both find peace and joy beyond them. Lile and Libby listen while I tell them all about trying new things like yoga and road trips and wine and they make me promise to call more often to keep them updated. Even my daddy's excited for me. I go to Los Angeles for an online marketing workshop, and when I'm there, walking down La Brea Boulevard with a new friend and talking about my separation, Daddy sends a snow-white feather to my feet. As it slow-falls down to the sun-bleached sidewalk, I time-travel back to childhood, sitting tucked under his arm in Grace Church, listening to him tell stories about our stained-glass dove.

Whenever you see the bird, know your daddy's thinking about you and that he loves you so much.

Jack is not excited. He's angry and I understand. I'm shocked when I hear from him on a very hot Tuesday in June and he wants to begin seeing our therapist, Jane, again. He seems to be done with me but for some reason—Jesus, maybe, or fear, or pride—he's unwilling to undo us completely, so we sit every week and sort through the hurts. It hurts when he sees me smiling, when I post pictures online of myself doing things with strangers that I never did with him. It hurts when he sees me rent out the upstairs of our big blue house to travelers and take care of them more lovingly than I could care for him. It hurts when I start calling myself "Ruthie Lindsey" again. I think it hurts the most when he sees me dancing. I wish he really knew that I would have given anything to be able to love him and dance with him back then, the way I can now. It's been a very long time since I danced with a man that way.

Liam is standing next to a wall of denim at my favorite boutique when we meet. He's wearing a T-shirt that looks very soft and his eyes are the same color that all the pants are. His beard is coarse and shiny, a mix of perplexing brown-black darkness, and I can feel him welcoming me closer to him, though he never actually says it with words. He's in town shooting a documentary about a semi-famous local artist named Percy and they're filming inside the store when I pop by to visit my friend John Christian, who works there. I jangle the door open. Liam crouches low to fiddle with his lens and something inside my body changes.

I've just come from the park, where I was picnicking with Katie and crying into the perfect, buzz-cut grass about the inevitability of divorce. My cheeks are salty and my hair is a mess and I stink like mayonnaise on hot ham sandwiches. John Christian is a new friend but a favorite one; he runs up to me in his bow tie and gingham shirt and he looks so adorable I could eat him up. His cheeks are flushed and he's grinning like a fox, looking pleased that I arrived just in time to meet the cute boys taking pictures in the back of his store. He's been telling me for weeks that a cute boy is exactly what I need.

"Ruthie!" he drawls. "You have to meet these cool guys."

He squeezes my hands, winks, and introduces us. The situation seems almost too satisfying for him to withstand.

Liam says my name one time in his low purr of a voice and I almost fall over.

My body has been a lot of things, but since childhood, it's never been a home. It's been a meeting place for pain and fear, a landfill where medicine and sugar decay into a black mush, a laboratory for therapists and surgeons and diets, a detention hall where shame bats a yardstick at desire. In my mind, it's been too fat, too skinny, and too broken. It's cried out for things, rest and love and sex, but I've never listened; I've bowed to other voices instead, to a church that told me to hide it behind a glass casement, not to dress it or let it dance in a way that would make men's bodies cry out for it, to doctors who instructed me to "manage it," feed it pills and plaster it with patches. Jack is the only man I've ever slept in a bed with or even imagined sleeping beside. Besides Jack, I'd never really dated, I've not drunk or done drugs, besides the few times I nervously tried some skunky weed in an attempt to alleviate my pain. At twenty-three, when we met, I was still a little girl clinging to her purity, recoiling from a world that seemed too harsh and scary. I'm not a little girl anymore. When I see Liam, my body speaks to me and I'm listening, to the hot blood in my cheeks, the tangle of nerves sitting in my chest, the wanting. He asks if I want to meet up later and again, I say yes.

We go to a dive bar in a double-wide near the fairgrounds called Santa's. There are too many people inside and all of them are smoking cigarettes. I can hardly breathe, nobody can, but somehow, most of them growl their way through karaoke. The tables look like they were stolen from a bingo hall and there are so many twinkle lights strung up and stuffed into the same power strip, I feel like I'm back on my Christmas set. I buy a shitty beer and I drink it fast because I'm nervous and I need my heart to slow down. Liam sits next to me all night. He just grins at me through his beard like a Wooly Willy toy, like he's keeping a secret about me that even I don't know yet. I have another drink, he has two, and we talk and talk. He reaches over to take a sip of my beer, letting his hand rest on top of mine for four thrilling seconds, and I just can't believe that this gorgeous, wonderful man wants to be near me too.

Flirtatious glue holds us together while everyone else is in shambles, spilling on themselves, slurring their words and singing their best Jefferson Airplane. He waits almost two hours to tell me the secret he's been keeping.

"Ruthie, my job is to meet people and document them. I've been doing it for years, loving it for years, and I'll continue to do it forever. I've never met anybody like you before."

Three college girls struggle along to "Somebody to Love." They've only heard the chorus before, so the rest is just giggling.

"You're an interesting mix. One part little girl, filled with joy and excitement, and one part old lady, filled with wisdom and knowledge, just rocking away on her front porch."

He sees me.

Everything hushes and I get pins and needles in my face. I've never felt less looked at and more looked into.

"Yes."

It's the only word I can say.

We spend the following week together. We listen to music and let it carry us around my kitchen until we collapse into a pile of red wine breath and laughter and kisses. I know that he's leaving, but I don't care. He touches my body like it's holy ground, with tenderness and reverence, tiptoeing across the shape of my side like he doesn't want to disturb it, only to witness the magic of cool air on my skin. Lovingly and carefully, he cradles my face in both his hands and just *looks*. We go on walks and watch sunsets and fool around in the big sleigh bed like teenagers. I hear my hands and my heart and my hips as they speak, and instead of letting them be drowned out, I give them my trust. There is no shame when I see him resting on Jack's old pillow, there's no shame when he holds my hand on the street, there's no shame when I feel myself wanting him. I never thought I could be attracted to another man, let another man sleep beside me in my bed, but I can, I allow myself to. I feel safe and seen.

My body may have broken parts, but I can love devotedly with it, I can celebrate, exult, and let myself be moved. I can overcome bare-naked, buzzing nerves in my side to get up and dance for just one more song. I learn in these long, stretched-out nights and tender quiet mornings with him that my body doesn't have to be a perfect place to be a sacred one. It still doesn't feel quite like a home, but it feels closer to one.

Liam leaves on a Tuesday. He goes to Texas or Oklahoma or one of the Carolinas. He kisses me on the forehead on the front steps of my house in the broad white daylight. I want to say something clever but I say thank you instead, and he kisses me one more time.

That night, I'm alone and Mrs. God comes to see me in a frantic thunderstorm. She makes marimba music on the gutters to wake me, and the neighbor's wind chimes go wild, slamming into the window and tangling together. I open my eyes to the emptiness of the bed, the little rumpled shadow that Liam left behind, soft and sunken into the sheets. I reach for it, and mysteriously, it's still warm. The tornado sirens start screaming their windy-weather song and I smile. All across the city, recent transplants will be scurrying to their safe places while those of us who know better will stay in bed, look out the window, and just listen for the refrain, the crashing and the booming, rain spilling from the sky to the ground.

A big old branch across the street falls and rapids flow against the sidewalk banks. I'm not scared. I feel safe now, safer than I ever have. The gusts whistle at the trees while they bend to pick up their leaves and the power lines spin like jump ropes, but still I'm not afraid. It gets louder and more intense, but I don't see destruction. I see creation, the baptism of the lawn and the bathing of the asphalt. I see everything differently now. My lips curl around the glass of water that Jack used to bring me and I rub the wrinkles out of the sheets in the spot he used to sleep in. Our last therapy session comes back to me, his angry remembrance of our love story.

"I never would have been with you if I wasn't in such a bad place when we met."

"I'm done rescuing you."

"You don't want me. You just want a baby. I'm a means to an end."

His truth hurt me so badly to hear that my brain got blurry. How could my truth be so different from his? I remember him adoring me. I remember our long, lazy afternoons in the sheets and wanting to start a family.

Mother Nature plays her instruments with everything she has now. It's theater: the lightning makes daytime at 1 a.m. and I clutch at my heart.

Oh, Jack.

A counselor friend told me once that she could tell if a marriage was going to work. Looking back on their lives together, if a couple could only see the relationship through the lens of loss and pain, then it was over. Jack and I don't see the same things when we look back—he doesn't see beauty, growth, or redemption. He just sees hurt, he hears what's screaming the loudest. Our marriage is over in all ways but paperwork. I can't change what he sees when he looks back at us, but maybe if we look deep enough into each other, he'll be able to look forward and find healing, peace. Maybe I will too.

19

Two Thousand Words

Jack's lips are quivering. His beard is longer and thicker and grayer than I've seen it before, than I ever thought it could be. If it weren't for the mouth, that shaky mouth that snores late at night and gets small when it's angry and gives long, thoughtful kisses, if I couldn't see it peeking through the salt-and-pepper terrier fur, I'd hardly recognize the only man I've ever loved. The air-conditioning roars as I walk into the room and little bits of late-July heat come with me. Jack's body shudders, a chill wiggles through him, and the love seat creaks underneath his hips. We've sat together on the little couch before, but this time he's in the middle and I have to find a separate space. Today is the last day, the last $150 check we write Jane, the very last moments of belonging to each other. Today, we will say goodbye.

Jane is shuffling around at her desk in the corner. I take her in one last time too. Even though it's ninety-five degrees outside, she's committed to a shawl the color of raw tuna, and it keeps getting caught up in the drawer handles. She smiles at me, flustered and a little sad. She's always seemed to like us. She pushes a deep breath out of her nose as she moves a pair of glasses high up on the bridge of it. Poor Jane, she knows that today is the last day too.

"Hi," I say to both of them, because nobody else has said anything at all.

I join them in the triangle of seats and settle into Jane's armchair, which I suspect is there specifically for couples like us, who don't want to be next to each other anymore. Jack looks up, he finds my face. His brownie-batter eyes are as bottomless and thoughtful and beautiful as they ever have been but they're so full of shame. They're deep, muddy pits in his face flanked by bloodshot membranes and blue-gray pillows of worry. I can feel how tired he is. The weight of every hour he's stayed awake wondering if there's another way, of every beer he's cracked before noon, of each word he's said to hurt me—it's all left him puffy and pale, like a grungy, half-melted snowman. Of all the days we've been together, today, the day of our undoing, is the day I want to hold him the most.

Jane says something kind about us working hard and being brave, but neither one of us responds. We just sit in silence together and quietly meditate on the past six months, deciding what love is and wondering if we have enough of it. He doesn't want to speak first, so out of mercy, I do.

"I can't live like this anymore. You're not going to come back— it's been months. You left me and you need to finish this. Please, Jack, just say that it's over."

He's a huge, lumbering, now heavily bearded man, but in this room, in this moment, he's freckle-faced and has fallen off his tricycle. I could pick him up and carry him away. The sun laser-beams through a big window behind him and raises sweat on the back of his neck. His eyes are fixed straight ahead at the noth-ingness on the wall, avoiding mine. Phlegm rumbles in his throat and he fidgets with his hands. He's always drumming, even if just in his imagination. The words are there but he can't get them out.

"Take your time," Jane says, and he does.

His lips still vibrate under his nose and I watch them, remem-bering all the other times they've done that before: the day he pro-posed down on one knee surrounded by Dollar Store candles and roses, the day he led me toward the stillness of my daddy's body, the morning they took me into surgery at Mayo and I thought he was going to chase after the gurney. The day that he left six months ago. I'm struck dumb by how well I know him, the way his face moves and the sound his breath makes. Those are parts of him I'll probably always know. I rewind a decade of loving each other and play it back to myself until I can't anymore.

"Please, Jack, I need you to say it."

Jane glares at me as much as someone who looks like Mother Goose can glare at you, but I ignore her. His eyes drop down and we look at each other; we look into each other, finally.

"I don't want to be married to you anymore. I'm going to file for divorce."

His head drops into his hands like a bowling ball and Jane qui-etly places a cube of Kleenex next to him on the sofa. I watch his fingers shake on his forehead and imagine all the things he must be telling himself:

You're a failure.

You're not a Christian.

You're giving up.

You're just like your dad.

223

I wonder if Jack knows that those stories aren't true, that they never have been.

There's a big, long, silent thinking that happens, and then I speak.

"Jane, will you leave us?"

She touches Jack's shoulder. "Is that okay?"

He nods. It feels strange when she asks for his permission, but I understand. She rises from her chair, straightens her shawl, and walks outside.

I have never been able to love Jack, not really, not the way he needed me to. When I walked toward him in that low-backed $250 bridesmaid's dress, I carried with me the promise of partnership, family, respite, and support, but what life delivered to us was so different from what we expected. There was no partnership. I was the ward and he was the keeper. I was the patient and he was the caretaker. I was a puzzle with too many missing pieces that for years he refused to put down. He was sick—probably the whole time—but my sickness dwarfed his. My life dwarfed our life. My desire to be a mother swallowed my desire to be his wife. I treated him like a sperm donor. Even still, through what had to be misery and anger, he showed up for me, he loved me as best he could for as long as he could. Today, in this room, where for months we've invited our anger to speak for us, it's just me and him, two people who will always know each other a little bit, who will be twisted together by memories, deep love and deep sorrow. For the very first and very last time, I love him the way I never could before.

I move from my chair to sit next to him and I pull his warm, weeping body into mine. I rock him and shush him like the child we never had together and I love him like the woman I hope he'll find one day. He melts into me and his hot-water tears drip down over my shoulders, I've been closer to him before, but I've never seen him so clearly as I do right now. I see all the goodness in him and all the grief; I see somebody who deserves healing and hope. I see so much beauty in him and I smile, it's a real smile.

"Jack, I'm so sorry. I'm so sorry I couldn't show up for you the way you showed up for me. I didn't know how to give you the love you needed. I didn't even know how to love myself. You're such a good man and I feel so lucky that it was you. I'm so happy that you were the one who was there for me. You're going to be an amazing husband to someone and an amazing dad. Everything's going to be okay."

I'm holding him up. His big body begins to bob and shake, and both of us wobble. The love seat groans under us like an old bed frame—it might tip over.

"You're so good, you're so kind, and you're so loved. I will never, ever speak ill of you. I'm so thankful for everything you've done."

I can hear Jane's shoes scraping across the drive outside. There's one more thing I need him to know.

"Jack, you're not your dad."

He pulls his bloated red face back from my chest and looks at me. He's so beautiful, so pure, and so loved. God is written all over him.

"I'm sorry too. You'll be a great mom one day and I hope you find somebody who can love you fully."

I just keep holding on to him and the tender ending of us until we run out of time.

Moving forward is peaceful but sad. I don't miss being married to Jack but I mourn the loss of him. We're getting divorced. The knowledge is hefty to lug around. He won't see our niece, Kitty, graduate high school and I'll never learn to fly-fish on the Colorado River like I said I would. When his parents get cancer, nobody will tell me.

I stay busy all summer working my body too hard on photo shoots, spending too much time on Instagram, and drinking. I'm a glutton. I cover up the hurt and confusion with whatever I can find that feels good, and eventually, I cover myself up completely. I convince myself that social media is an inventory of my blessings, but just like my bed, it becomes another comfortable place to hide. Every year since the surgery at Mayo, my pain has gotten worse; every day since Jack left, my heart has felt empty. Instead of honoring my pain, sharing it, I detach, disconnect, and refuse to let my world be anything but skies of melted sherbet, seven different kinds of wildflowers in my grandma's milk-glass vases, and friendships. The silence hurts, so I make as much noise as I can. My body hurts, so I hang stylish clothing on it, keep it busy, and take pictures. At thirty-four years old, I'm still performing for company, my thousands of followers, like a gangly little girl. Beauty and adoration are effective medicines and I consume, consume, consume, cutting flowers from the bushes I pass, having another taco, another drink, buying this and that. I cover everything that hurts with anything that doesn't. I know that you can't treat the wound unless you let it breathe. Defiantly, I try to smother it.

When I wake up, my mouth is dry and tarry from secondhand smoke and my nighttime makeup is curdled gunk on my cheeks. It's August 2013. Amber took me dancing and drinking last night.

I'm dehydrated and my muscles are tight and angry. It's only 5:15 a.m. but pain is an early riser, so God's morning sky gets the audience it deserves in me and the chatty brown birds outside. I swing my legs over the side of the bed and the nerves clench together into a ball on my back when the weight of me sinks to the floor. I grab onto the bed, holding myself up with a handful of sheet, and wonder how many more years I'll be able to dance, or walk, or live alone. The countdown to frailty has already begun. Still woozy, I hear ticking and tocking in my temples.

Broad, aching waves radiate up my spine as I walk to the kitchen for water. The lights are too bright but I'm not strong enough, steady enough, or willing enough to go to the switch across the room. I lean over the counter, smack the faucet on, and lift the glass to my lips, letting its contents spill all over and into the fancy apron sink we paid extra for. The shuffle back to the bedroom is slow and humiliating; the too-bright lights and chirpy birds blink and snicker at me from the branches outside.

A sadness settles in during the three-minute climb from the floor to the bed and I grab for my phone. I need to see something different, something sweet and beautiful, so I open up my Instagram. Amber and I are tipsy in the pictures. I must have posted them last night. Our hair is suspended in the air, our mouths are stretched wide open, and our limbs are too fast-moving and fuzzy to be anything but swipes of pale pink. There are twenty-two comments already.

"I want your life."
"What a dream."
"You're so beautiful."
"I wish I was there!"

Another big, aching wave hits. I shut my eyes hard, grab onto my heating pad, and wait for it to pass over me. It never quite does though. I read the next one and clamp my molars together.

"Can we trade places?"

I feel sick. Don't they know?

Don't they know that I suffer? That I hurt and ache and grieve? Don't they know?

I swipe back through my cheerful daisy chain of pictures. There I am, smiling big and saying nothing. I'm pretty and fun and happy all the time. I'm hiding.

The scar that runs up my spine is soft and pink. It climbs up my neck completely concealed by an undercoat of curly hair that never grew back in right. Everything that hurts is hidden. It's always been that way: scars that slide effortlessly under clothing, dependencies legitimized by prescriptions, duty disguised as marriage. I reach back and run my hand up to find the place where new skin meets old.

I'm tired of hiding.

I lie awake on my back for hours, thinking and hurting and letting a strange energy speak to me. I think about the community I've assembled on social media who really don't know me, who I don't really let know me. I think about the stories I choose to tell them and the ones that I don't. I remember 2010. I spent almost the entire year lying in my bed, eyes glassy from too much Facebook: pregnant bellies; couples in love; perfect, fit, pain-free bodies. It made me miserable. Now, as I curate, collect, and cover pain with beauty to make myself feel better, I know I could be making someone else feel worse. I've meant every beautiful word I've shared with the world, but there are so many other words that

I haven't shared. I haven't shared my pain, even though I know that pain is universal, relatable, and real. Everybody knows hurt and loss, but I've only shared the prettiest pictures of my life, the images and stories that hurt the least for me to look at.

At 12:45 p.m., six glasses of water, two ibuprofen, and one muffin into my day, I go to the pour-over-coffee place where I like to work and I stop hiding my pain. I tell my story, knowing that there are ugly parts, knowing that there's pain, but also knowing that there's dignity and power and beauty in my story. I decide to stop worrying about pushing people away with the not-so-pretty parts of life, to stop selling them short. To stop selling myself short.

I write about the accident.

"When I was a senior in high school, I was in a terrible car accident. I broke three ribs, which then punctured my lungs. As a result, they collapsed, my spleen ruptured, and I broke the top two vertebrae in my spine. . . ."

I write about the wire and the drugs.

". . . the pain continued to get worse and worse, to the point that I needed narcotics to help me cope. I felt desperate and fearful for my life."

I write about Jack.

"I have so much empathy for the man who's been my husband. I can't even imagine what it was like on his end to get married at twenty-two and to be dealt the cards we were—parents divorcing, a wife with chronic pain who dealt with it very poorly, a father-in-law's death, the financial burden of medical bills, and a struggle with infertility."

I tell the truth about who I am and why I'm here.

"To be where I am now is not at all what I envisioned for myself. But my life is rich and lovely. I feel tenderness and mercy surrounding me every day, and I try to hold on to it tight. I share all of this with you because I feel like my purpose is to share the story of living a beautiful and rich life in the midst of heartache and pain."

I type like I dance: clumsily, loudly, and from the depths of me. The polite coffee shop people negotiate their too-tall biscuits that drip with bright orange egg yolk and look curiously at me. I read it over just once, while the music of dirty dishes tumbling into a rubber bin behind me plays over and over. I hit "publish" and something so heavy is lifted away from me.

The internet normally prefers short stories, but my story is not short or pretty or simple. It's two thousand messy, honest, triumphant words that go viral. In the months that follow, I write more and take fewer pictures. I unlearn the stories I told myself about perfection and replace them with new stories about wholeness, about beauty *and* pain, joy *and* suffering. The pain that nearly killed me brings me to life. Pain becomes as much a part of my mission as beauty is.

Just like when I was a little girl, I feel beloved, the luckiest of the lucky. It's what I've always wanted. The light that comes at me from the outside becomes so big and so bright that I bask in it, let myself be nurtured by it and forget about the inside of me. My pain grows louder and louder but so does my life. When life gets too loud, it becomes very hard to listen. I still have to fight for glimpses of myself.

20

Human Energy Sponge

The water in Nicaragua is stained glass. It glows phosphorescent and casts light over my broken body, which is gently held by the salty water. I smile—it looks like the ocean is filled with fireflies and it reminds me of home, of sitting on our farm and watching them flicker and dance through the evening. Venus appears above and the weight of my broken body lifts from me. I feel safe as I float across the bay, like I'm tucked into the pew at Grace Church next to my daddy.

It's my first time in Central America. I'm not alone here. There are other bodies sloshing around beside me in the blue glitter. I'm here to help promote a beautiful surfing village, to style photos and write about it on Instagram. I can't surf, but nobody seems to mind. I fall in love with the people here quickly. It seems totally wild to me, but since my story started spreading on the internet, I get to go on adventures like these often. Companies send me clothes to wear and lend me cars to drive on road trips. I'm kind of in marketing, kind of a writer (if long-winded Instagram posts

RUTHIE LINDSEY

count), kind of a stylist, kind of a lot of things. I feel like I'm tricking people. I don't really know what I'm doing, but they seem to like me and it still feels good to be loved that way.

The little algae hang on to my body as I let the water carry me around like I'm a favorite rag doll. The sound of sea-foam creeping onto the powdery white beach brings me peace and I close my eyes. Everything becomes still.

I have to brace myself for the stillness. My body is suffering and I don't take much time to converse with it. The things it has to say are not always easy to hear. It cries to me.

I'm hurting.

I'm so tired.

Please listen.

Most days, it's easier to keep it moving, keep myself distracted, than it is to stop and listen.

"Ruthie!" somebody howls out from the shore.

I need rest.

"Ruuuuuthieeeeeee!"

The giggles are sloppy and lager soaked, filled with the promise of a good time.

We need to talk.

But I can't. Not right now.

I let the jungle drown the quiet voice inside me with its bugs and frogs and howler monkeys, who are as small as cats but sound like dinosaurs. I drag my arms through the water toward the beautiful people waiting for me in this beautiful place. My world has gotten bigger and louder. It's been easy to lose myself in it.

My story keeps traveling and I travel along with it, to Canada and Belgium and Mexico and France. I go as far from home as my story will take me, and I get filled up by the new places and faces and skylines. I keep staying true to the choice I made. Instead of staying in my bed and hurting, I serve and hurt, live and hurt, learn and hurt. I meet amazing people and lots of new friends, many of whom don't speak my language, look like me, or live like me, and it feels like the greatest gift. I say yes over and over, to opportunities that thrill, scare, and move me. I learn the importance of community, of surrounding myself with people who inspire me and act as my teachers here in earth school, people who tell the truth and push me closer toward mine. One of them is called Jed.

There is nobody else like Jedidiah Jenkins. We met through Instagram while he was biking from Oregon to Patagonia, and one day, after his journey was over, he just showed up at my door in Nashville. It felt like a missing piece of my heart showed up and jumped back into my chest. Jed is a writer and an adventurer. He knows all the plants and birds and sees things in intricate detail that I don't even notice. He wants to watch people from a distance, and I want to scoop them up in my arms. He shares earnestly with his following, stripping layer after layer away from himself; I clamor around for extra scraps of protection. We're different, staggeringly so.

In 2015, companies begin hiring us to speak and travel together. We make silly videos and sing. We laugh when the internet ignores the fact that Jed is gay and asks when we'll have babies. We road-trip across the country from event to event and I try to do it all with a smile on my face. Jed doesn't smile unless he wants to. We're together all the time and he really sees me, the masks I need to wear to get through the day, or the job, or the next hundred miles of highway. He's one of the first people to notice the impact this life I'm leading is having on me, watching with concerned eyes as my body fails me, and even more so as I fail my body. He watches me push too hard, pick myself up, and keep pretending.

"You don't have to do this," he tells me as we chat about the next gig.

But I just keep going, curling up in our hotel room at the end of the night on my heating pad and thinking about truth. Jed doesn't wear a mask. He writes about his flaws, his pain, his God, his deepest, darkest feelings, without a single apology. He knows himself. I begin to realize that I've barely begun to learn who I am.

"Ruthie is a human energy sponge," he writes on Instagram one day. *"She feels the room. She walks in and knows exactly who has had a bad day, who just fought with their girlfriend, and who feels inadequate."*

I'm good at absorbing the pain of others, at serving them and showing up for them. But I know that at some point I'll have to show up for myself.

The farther I travel, the longer it all goes on, the more I feel like a sponge—heavy, moldy, dripping wet, desperate to be wrung out or thrown away.

Over the next two years, magazines and blogs begin to interview me. I notice that pain is at the center of every conversation, every presentation. I talk about the accident, about losing my daddy, losing Jack, and weaning myself off pain meds. I talk about choosing joy, about the gifts that pain gave me. I'm softer, more empathetic. I don't want to be bitter and I don't feel that pain and divorce have to make a person that way, but we get to choose. My pain becomes a vehicle to help people, to serve them and bring them hope. The purpose it brings feels good to me, as close to a calling as I've ever known. I jump into helping people, I pour my soul into it, but I do so at a great cost. I have to sneak away during jobs to lie down with my heating pad. I occasionally drink too much at night to quiet the red ants, and when I get home I crash mightily for days at a time. Sometimes I get physically ill from the sheer intensity of the pain and the pace of life. I talk about hope, but sometimes I don't really have much. I'm terrified of the future and I believe that my pain will only get worse. I numb fear with noise the same way I numb the pain, hopping from fix to fix, distraction to distraction.

My body keeps speaking to me as I cram it into another economy airline seat, perch it behind another podium, fill it with junk food and Malbec.

I need you to slow down.

I need you to breathe.

I need you to listen to me.

But I drown it out with what's bright and beautiful and busy. I show up, but I pay the price.

My pain intensifies as I go and go. It becomes more grating and less forgiving. My nerve damage feels extensive but I stay away from doctors and pills and try to "manage it" on my own. Everywhere I go, I take the red ants along with me. They march up and down my side as I travel and write and sleep, as I dance and meet new people and date for the first time, as I embrace my sexuality instead of quieting it with shame. I dull my pain by denying it, defying it, not letting it slow me down. Serving others brings in the love and affirmation, but I lean on it, and as time goes on I become less capable of loving myself. I have to disconnect—let my mind and spirit stray from my pain so that it doesn't consume me, so that I can keep up with the beautiful life I've built for myself, a life that begins to fall apart.

I go to Big Bear in February 2017. It's a blanket of fat golden trees and gorgeous lakes in the middle of the San Bernardino Mountains. They hold a wildly popular photography conference there and they hired me to speak, even though I don't own a camera. They tell me they're diversifying this year, bringing in a wellness component, they want to tell new stories. My story doesn't feel new anymore, it feels as old and tired as my body, but I go anyway.

I don't feel well when I get off the plane at LAX. The pain got the best of me thirty-five thousand feet over Texas and it's stuck around. I haul my big plastic suitcase behind me through the terminal and look around at all the people careening carelessly, drunk on their phones. Their busy eyes, pink and brown and black faces, old and young, all pointed down—CNN, Facebook, the time, Amazon, anything that feels good. I smile big at them but nobody smiles back. People make less and less time to see each other these days. I'm sad about it, but I'm complicit. I do it too. My phone is a new drug and it's a powerful one. I have beauty, brightness, and "love" at my fingertips twenty-four hours a day. I can't put it down.

"They say it might snow up there," the white-haired lady at the Avis counter whispers at me, as though snow in the mountains is a secret just between us.

"I hope so," I say back to her. I have to force the friendliness; my body is screaming at me. I want to be alone.

She hands me the keys to a tiny rental car and waves.

"Be safe."

"I will," I promise her. But nothing feels safe.

The drive takes two hours. I listen to Matt Corby the entire time, rising up from the starving, gray desert, through the mist of low-hanging clouds, to the base of the powder-capped mountains. The altitude makes my temples twitch angrily at me—another migraine.

I clutch the wheel as my little car skids and I make my way around a big mound of mossy rock. The road becomes a spiraling Slinky, taking me round and round. The pain nags at me and I want to go home. With each turn, I look to the sky and pray the same way I did back in Libby's garden.

Make it be beautiful. Make it be beautiful. Make it be beautiful.

After the hundredth bend in the road, the sky changes. The sun has sunk somewhere below me and left a radiant spill of raspberry pink and orange and buttercup yellow. I pull onto a wide shoulder that must be especially for sky watching, and step out into the air. It's twenty degrees cooler than I thought it would be.

"Look at that sky!"

I take a picture and look at the sunset. I focus on the beauty and wait for the relief. My muscles go slack; everything hurts a little bit less. The colors ebb and flow and then vanish completely. The beauty pauses the pain for a moment—it distracts me, but it never lasts.

I arrive at the venue by nightfall and all anyone can talk about is snow. The outdoorsy Patagonia-vest types can hardly contain their excitement as they pace through the lodge and ready their lenses for the perfect picture. My body is ready for bed but I know how it will feel when I lay it down for rest; the red ants will take over, the migraine will come back. I just can't bear the idea of stillness right now, so I stay up, stretching my eyes and my smile wide and waiting by the windows with the others. We drink dark-colored drinks and laugh and make the beginnings of friendships. The snow never happens but nobody seems to care. At around 2 a.m., we all slip away to bed.

My talk is in room 4B the next morning. Pain rises with the sun to settle up with me, collect the cost of last night's fun. I didn't sleep well, but I hardly ever do. I have to lie faceup like I'm on an embalming table just to get close to comfortable. Sometimes, sleep takes hours to come. Sometimes, sleep doesn't come at all. My neck and back scream at me when I try to rest and my mind races. I think about how badly I'm hurting, how badly I *will* hurt when I'm fifty, seventy, eighty years old. I don't want to get old. I've accepted my pain and I wouldn't change it. I have deep gratitude for the new eyes it's given me to see people, the new arms to reach them, but pain also scares me. Sometimes I say yes because I want to; other times I say it because there's an urgency, a knowing that one day, I won't be able to zip-line in Vermont or travel to Europe. After a long night of spinning my wheels and watching the cobwebs sway, I feel exhausted by a future that hasn't arrived yet.

The lodge is wild when I go downstairs, bodies bumping into bodies. There's palpable excitement. People rush by me, staring at their screens and fast-walking to the places they're supposed to be.

A redheaded girl takes a video of herself by the middle of the doorway and I wait. She adjusts the angle of her chin and pats her hair a little. I wonder how many times I've been too busy to notice another body next to mine, how many times I've been too busy to notice my own body. I smile big at her when she's done and walk through the threshold.

Room 4B looks like the inside of an Apple store. There are about thirty to forty millennials, a herd made up of shutterbugs and artfully dressed-down hipsters, a few people I recognize from the night before. I wave at them and take it all in. The chairs are arranged in a giant sing-along circle that's probably supposed to create intimacy but mostly just creates a giant awkward space to stare into while I talk. I open my mouth to begin, but my body speaks first.

I feel really horrible.

A migraine hits. The red ants crawl up and down.

I need a break.

I clear my throat, push the voice away, and force my grin further. I look out into the sea of the thick-rimmed glasses and happy faces and wonder if anyone else is forcing it too.

I say the words I always do and hear them softly bounce off the shiny varnished ceilings. I see nods of approval, brows furrowed in concentration, recognition, affirmation. It makes the pain feel a little more distant, for now.

Outside, a few feathery tufts of snow drop down from the clouds: a late but welcome arrival. The sight disarms me, and silently we watch it out the window tumbling and settling onto the ground.

Suddenly, in the moment of stillness, I feel my daddy with me. I see his joyful, mischief-filled eyes, I remember the weight of his hand on mine, playing games on the drive home from school. Grief hits hard.

I try to speak through it, stick to the script that I know: pain, beauty, etc., but the words get caught in my throat.

A catastrophic tremor climbs up my side and my body speaks again.

Stop.

Rest.

I need you.

And this time, I do stop. I have to. I'm ragged and aching and I miss my daddy. I sink deep into my chair, stare out into the flannel hipster ocean, and start to cry.

"Sorry, I feel really terrible. This is hard," I tell them.

The room starts to cry along with me in big, fat sniffly tears. I'm not sure I know why, or if they do, but we just sit there and unravel together. I can't keep this up forever. Even on the top of a mountain surrounded by the incredible beauty, the pain is debilitating. We get quiet, we get still, and my body says something new.

Thank you.

I talk a little longer. I'm more raw and more truthful than I've ever been, more exposed. They don't shy away from the honesty, and the connection I feel to them feels different than normal, more beautiful, and wholly pure. When I'm done, I stand up, walk out into the big empty space they gave to me, and do something new. I hold each of their faces in my hands and speak to them one by one.

"Thank you," I say to them. "You are so loved. You are so needed. There is so much hope for you."

Afterward, they all walk up to me, shyly and sweetly, and do the same. It feels so good to have the words said back to me. I know they're true for others, but I struggle to tell them to myself and actually believe them. I believe them today. The love I feel as their hands gently graze my face is deep and nurturing. It takes me straight back to my mother's arms at five years old. This is community, this is love.

There, in room 4B, I catch a glimpse of myself: safe, smiling, and whole. I don't want to let go of it, but it fades as the pain comes crawling up my side.

A girl from Portland gives me stretchy gold pants to wear and paints glitter on my face. There's a dress-up party tonight to close out the weekend. I didn't bring anything to wear, but I would go naked if I had to: there's going to be dancing. When I'm dancing I see myself best, where the truest joy exists for me. I want to get another glimpse again.

The room is a pitch-black cave filled with flashing Technicolor rainbow lights and puffs of dry-ice smoke. I feel too old to be here, too grown-up, but I don't care: they're playing all my favorite songs— "No Diggity," "Regulate," and "Shoop." I take my shoes off the way I always do and dance with furious bliss, watching the way my arms move frame by frame by frame through neon sheets of color and light, letting the reverberations from the speakers blow over me like a breeze. My heart beats fast. My muscles seize up. The pain is deep and heavy. I try to shake it off, try to defy it. I twist and I bend and I don't let it win. I escape into the movement and the music.

They're serving alcohol but I don't want it, I don't need it. There are men here, sidling up to me slowly, spinning me around, flirting. I don't want them either. I just want to dance. I just want to feel good. I don't want to hurt anymore.

The room gets too loud and too crowded. There are too many colors and voices and I feel a pain rise up at the base of my neck and swell over my entire skull. My body speaks to me.

It's time to go.

It's time to rest.

I refuse to listen, to let pain rob me of the joy again. I won't go until I get my glimpse. I leave the big hall and I go to find a new space for myself.

The music travels through the walls and makes the stock art rattle in its frames. I dance down a long, strange hallway that snakes to the back of the building. There's an empty room, a place where nobody really goes. The nighttime lights are on and the floor is dirty. The soles of my feet are black, covered in filth and crumbs and spilled drink, but I don't care. I close my eyes and I start to sway, music buzzing in my feet, up my legs, landing in the middle of my chest. I twirl around and around.

Stop, my body pleads, but again, I refuse.

I want one dance that belongs only to me, not to pain, not a performance for anybody else. I want to feel young, free, and unburdened. Salty little beads teardrop down the back of my neck as I move, clinging to the creaminess of my scars and shooting down the hollow of my spine. The borrowed clothes are soaking wet, they stink, but I don't care. Snow comes down in dove-colored tufts outside and my feet move faster as the snowflakes multiply and become a thick, cloudy blizzard. As the moon sends its silvery glow slinking into the room, I see her—my spirit, my highest loving self. She's so good and so whole and I let her lead me around the room.

My body dances without thought or instruction. As I twist and let myself be moved by my loving spirit, she speaks to me.

She asks me to stop ignoring her, to allow myself to feel beautiful, to stop calling myself broken. I speak so often about self-love, but the things I tell myself aren't loving: *No man will be able to handle your pain, you'll be alone forever.* The beliefs are so limiting, and I finally begin to see that as she extends an invitation not to dance anything away, but to dance through what I feel. I cry full, earnest tears as I sway and embrace what I normally push down: rage, frustration, grief, and sadness. By the end, the dirty room is a holy place. I'm feeling love and compassion for myself. I'm feeling beautiful and worthy. Soaking wet and sobbing as I walk back down the empty hallway, I know I want to feel those things as much as possible.

When I get home to Nashville, the pain is worse than I knew it could be, but there's the promise of true and deep love inside myself. I lay my weapons down. I decide I want to make peace with pain, and I begin a healing journey.

21

Journeying

"This is my best friend Ruthie Ru. She's so courageous, so loving. She's such a loyal and true friend. I'm in awe of her perseverance and determination."

There are nine other people in the room and I can feel my pulse up the side of my neck. It's early spring. The air is sweet, not too humid yet, and everything's about to start blooming. I look out at the group, all different ages and stages of life, all here for different reasons. Our counselor, Barbara, whom we lovingly call "Babs," is standing beside me smiling warmly. We just met, but I feel like she's known me for years. She feels safe and wise and I trust her immediately.

It's our first group session. To start, Babs takes us through a meditation to help us identify one of the people in our lives we feel loves us the deepest. Then she asks us to introduce ourselves through that person's eyes. I choose Katie—she's always seemed to see me better than I could see myself. She's loved me for twenty years, through my marriage, through my pain, through all of it.

She laid next to me in my bed when I had *C. diff* and couldn't stop shitting my pants.

The group smiles and says hello to me and I sit back down in the circle as a sweet man in his late seventies introduces himself through the eyes of his seven-year-old granddaughter and we all fall apart.

Onsite is a giant green expanse filled with the best-looking horses eating the best-looking grass you've ever seen. It isn't a treatment center, it's an emotional wellness center that offers therapeutic and personal growth workshops. They have experiential therapy programs for all kinds of things. Mine is called Living Centered and it's designed to help participants bring their lives back to center and to enhance emotional health. Mostly, Onsite is a safe place to take off your mask. I've been wearing mine for a very long time.

I came here to confront my pain and unlearn the story I've been telling myself: *You'll never get better, you are your pain, pain is your purpose.* Beyond the character in that story, the girl who can smile through agony and writes on the internet, I don't know who I am. All I get are glimpses.

The main dining hall is a Victorian mansion that looks like it was plucked straight from an *Anne of Green Gables* book. It has twinkle lights strung up along the eaves and rocking chairs. I keep expecting to see pies appear cooling on the window ledges but I'm pretty sure the chef is cooking gluten-free. I'm staying in a cabin a few steps away with two other women, one short and one tall. We're friendly, but we don't say much to each other. When you spend all day acting out your deepest traumas, there isn't much left to say. Onsite is exhausting, it's painful, and it's enlightening.

On the first day of treatment, they take our phones. My phone has been my lifeline. It was the first tool I had through which to start talking about pain. It was what I used to launch my career as a designer, the window I peeked through to see the world when I lived in my bed. It's the place I go to feel loved and affirmed. When I take it out of my bag and hand it over to the nice man with the safe-deposit box, I panic a little. I'm sad that I'll miss the premiere of Kendrick Lamar's new video. I don't know what I'll do without podcasts or shows to watch when pain keeps me up at night. My phone helps me escape and I'm nervous not to have it. I feel like I'm giving away a limb to somebody I don't even know.

We also aren't allowed to talk about what we do for a living. Babs doesn't care if you're a CEO or an Uber driver or an elephant, she cares about how connected you are to your soul, that you know your inherent worth to the world that you live in. Here, they say people tend to live like "human doings" instead of human beings, that we attach too much worth to our careers and the careers of others. Those things don't have anything to do with who we are on the inside, and Onsite is all about who you are inside. They put us through meditation exercises and acting exercises and exercises where you can beat the shit out of a giant foam square to get your anger and rage out in a safe space; they say our hysterical reactions are always historical, from pain and loss that have never been worked through or processed. I've been through a lot. I don't think focusing on who I am for a week will be difficult, but it is.

I knew that I found identity in my pain story when I lived in my bed. I liked the sympathy I got and the attention. I didn't know that it was still so deeply ingrained. I'm used to introducing myself as a speaker and I'm used to being asked what it is that I speak about. Typically, I give a compelling, five-minute overview of my life story: accident, pain, a mountain of medications, divorce, and typically I'm applauded for my bravery, for "overcoming" such intense pain. With no career to talk about at Onsite, all I have left is pain. It feels like the most important thing about me and I don't know who I am outside of it. I wonder if it's a crutch, if I'd have a career at all without it, if people would like me without it. The thoughts scare me. Through every exercise, every meal, every conversation, I try to connect without pain, I try to keep it at a distance and focus on who I am, but I don't know who that is. I talk about my pain to anyone who'll listen, and even after days of intense emotional work, the first thing I do when I wake up in the morning is ask myself how I can use pain to reach people, as though it's the only way I can. Our teacher encourages us to be the love inside us, to feel it from inside ourselves instead of looking outward. I wonder if without pain, that love exists for me.

Over the next year, I continue my deep dive into healing work. I look to every resource, therapy, and treatment to help keep pain standing beside me and point me in the direction of my new story. A glutton through and through, I try everything. I do neurofeedback and Reiki. I read Eckhart Tolle and Richard Rohr. I buy the purple amethyst crystal to feel clarity, the rose quartz to feel love, the black tourmaline to feel safe. I also get laser hair removal, which is totally unrelated but feels healing at the time. I get new tattoos and talk to mediums on the phone. I stay open and I welcome change. I do the work and wait for the sky to open and drop my intention at my feet. When that doesn't happen, I work harder, dive deeper. I try to make healing busy and loud because it's what I know to do. I consume more and more, look further and further for the answers—yoga videos, retreats, a sound bath, a dance class. I move wildly through all of it. My physical pain continues to intensify. The glimpses of my true self become more distant. Still, I keep moving, keep working, speaking at events and traveling for brands. Until I collapse.

Michelle sends me a message over Instagram. We worked at Camp DeSoto together but haven't spoken since. I remember her big smile and long, sinewy teenage body running around next to mine as we cut through the steam that rose off the lake in the morning. I remember her from the worship rocks. She grew from being a camp counselor with a whistle to an actual counselor with a downtown office in Nashville and she thinks that she can help me. Michelle performs something called "holotropic breathwork," a type of therapy focused deeply on the act of controlling one's breathing patterns to influence mental, emotional, and physical states for healing. She says it can help people with trauma. I'm unfamiliar with this treatment but I'm desperate, and when someone wants to help fix me, I still can't help but let them try.

I go to her office on a Tuesday and lie on the floor. The music she plays seems too loud for what we're doing. The sunlight is aggressive; it pushes through the long, stiff planks of curtain like they're made of tissue paper and makes my whole body sweat. The walls are barren. I sense this is on purpose but I don't know the reason why.

Michelle sits next to me on the tile, her legs crossed, and looking mostly the same as she did at eighteen. She asks me to scan my body.

It's miserable. I want to get up and leave but I don't. I start at my toes; my right foot is screaming at me, twisted nerves that echo and swell but never stop completely. At my ankle, the pain turns to heat; the red ants march from the back of my leg to the back of my skull.

My mind speaks to me. *Everything's okay. Everything's okay. Everything's okay.*

My body speaks. *No, it isn't. No, it isn't. No, it isn't.*

I think it as hard as I can while the pain becomes as loud and unruly and strange as the music. I keep working my way up, up, up, winding past the mounds of white flesh left over from where they took bone from my hip to repair my neck after the accident. I travel to my ribs, my lungs, my guts, I take an inventory of tired bones and missing pieces.

Michelle is a loving presence. For fifteen minutes, she's just with me as I take deep breaths. She doesn't say anything; she just watches my body fill with the awareness it tries so hard to avoid.

"Now, Ruthie"—she's gentle when she asks—"tell me how you're feeling."

"My feet are frozen, my lips are chapped, my throat is dry, and I'm cold."

She uncurls her long legs and brings me everything I need: a crocheted blanket with perfect toe-shaped holes for my feet, my ChapStick, and a bottle of water.

I lie back down covered in a confusing mix of sweat and goose bumps. I know I'm wasting her time. She can't help me with inhales and exhales, I've tried that. I've tried everything. I'm unfixable, totally disconnected from my body. She speaks again like she can hear me spiraling over the drums thumping out of her little speakers in the corner.

"Open up your mouth wide and breathe as deeply as you can."

The breath comes out of me hot and ragged; my jaw is cranked down to my chest. I do this for what seems like forever but is probably only a few minutes. I feel so awkward and uncomfortable and am sure this won't work for me.

"Now, tap along to the music," she then says.

I press my fingertips into the floor softly at first, picking up little pebbles and hairs and bits of dirt, but I start to go faster and harder, catching up to the chaos of the song. My eyelids smash together and the room shrinks.

Bam! Bam! Bam!

I'm slapping the floor now. Fat and salty tears slide down onto my neck. Michelle places Kleenex on my cheeks and asks if she can put her hands on my heart. I say yes.

Bam! Bam! Bam!

My mind drifts into a strange half-awake dream space.

Someone approaches me in the fog. I recognize her voice right away.

"Hello, sweet Ruthie."

I see her. She's me, a perfect mirror version, my daddy's nose and my mom's big lashes, my long body and my dark mess of hair. Every scar and blemish is as alive on her skin as it is on mine but she's covered them with light and love and mercy. I look into her light-filled eyes: she's my truth, my divinity, my highest loving self.

She tilts my chin up to hers. "Can I show you something?"

I nod and let her lead me through the darkness.

We meet in the ICU at Baton Rouge General. It's 1996. My wrists are bound to the bed and I'm on life support. There's a tube in my throat and I can't speak.

She places one hand on her chest and one hand on mine, creating a link from heart to heart. My breath is rough and shallow but she begins taking deep, peaceful, healing breaths, and I follow her. We inhale and exhale in tandem and the panic turns to calmness.

"You will walk again and dance again. You're safe, you're so brave, and you'll have a beautiful life. I'm always here with you. I'll never leave you. I love you, sweet girl, and I'm so proud of you," she whispers.

I let her lead me onward.

I'm waking up from surgery at Mayo and the pain is unfathomable. I wish they would sedate me, that I could just check out of my body. She sits by the bed and my daddy appears for both of us. He smiles his beautiful, silly smile and covers us both in comfort. He grabs my fingers the way he used to in the car on the way to school, hands hard from the garden, hot from the sun, and I glow with comfort at seeing him again—we both do. He gently pats the coldness of my arm.

"Pat, pat, rub, rub. God loves you, Daddy loves you."

The strength we need comes to us through him.

We keep wandering.

The resident is trying to insert the spinal tap. The room is all stainless-steel instruments and nurses in flimsy light-blue uniforms holding me down. My family isn't here with me, it's just the medical staff, they're talking at me and touching me but not listening. They insist that everything's okay, but it isn't. My screams hit the ceiling but nobody seems to notice. The resident keeps stabbing into me again and again.

Her voice is low but demanding.

"Take your hands off my Ruthie. Do not touch her again."

She comes to me, shows up for me when nobody else can.

The doctor takes his hands off me, the nurses back away, scrubs swishing softly together, and they make space for her. She walks toward me as the gang dissolves, lifts me from the bed into her arms. My neck brace groans as I bury my head into the safety and protection of her shoulder and she carries me away.

We travel to the bathroom floor in the pretty yellow house. I'm curled into a ball staring into the white, empty window of a negative pregnancy test through tears that rise in my eyes faster than they can fall. The familiar cramps have already begun, the monthly hunger pangs of an empty womb. She brings my body into hers and holds me while I weep.

"Oh, beautiful soul! I know this is so hard, I'm so sorry, but dear Ruthie, you are a mother and you will get to mother so many in this life," she whispers.

She takes my hand again. "This will hurt, but you're ready."

My mind and body are coming undone: I'm in Little Lile's room wide awake at 3 a.m., staring at the Tiger clock as it stares back at me, begging myself to fall asleep and forget to wake up. She appears again. She lies down next to me and sings me to sleep with the sweetest songs; she holds my shaking body still and re-minds me, "You're not alone. I'm here for you—I'm inside you and around you and I always will be. You are never alone."

I blink at her with my wide, exhausted eyes.

"You're not broken, you are whole. Healing and hope are for you; a full and joyful life is for you."

We return to so many moments, so many traumas and hurts I've tried to erase. We handle each one with tenderness, covering it in love and mercy, leaving the most sacred scars. We unravel my traumatic stories and write new ones; we retell them with kindness and grace.

Before she leaves, we travel one last time. We go back to the big blue house. My marriage is ending. Jack is sitting across from me on the couch, eyes dry and distant. She sits next to him. His face warms when he feels her there and he smiles. She begins to speak to him for me.

"Jack, I wanted a baby more than I wanted you. I'm so sorry. You are a good man. You will be a husband and a father and you are worthy of the truest, most abundant, profound love. Don't carry this ending as shame; let it instead be a peace that lifts you."

They walk to the front door and stand in an embrace for a long time, staring and smiling and holding lovingly on to each other. She squeezes him tight and releases him. He walks outside.

I watch the door shut slowly behind him and walk into her open arms. We sway together under the sky-high ceilings.

"I know it hurts, but this pain will be what releases you, what cracks you open and makes space for joy and healing and purpose. You're going to help people, my sweet girl. Remember, you are love."

Her warm skin brushes up to mine as she cradles my face in her hands and looks at me with the most tender, compassionate eyes. We say it together as an affirmation:

"I am not broken, I am whole, I am loved, I am love."

Then she leaves me, but I don't feel alone at all.

A future I've been afraid to imagine unfolds in the strange, dreamy space. The ability to heal and comfort and love myself becomes clear, and I can see the joyful life it will bring:

I'm going to heal.

I will have a partner one day.

I'm worthy.

I can feel the Divine with me. It doesn't feel like Mrs. God anymore, just "the Divine," an energy, eternal, radical love. My soul feels closer to me than my pain does, and when I wake up, it still feels close. I don't have to look for glimpses of myself anymore. My highest self shows up for me. For the first time, I see the love and divinity that exist and have always existed inside me.

Michelle is still sitting next to me.

"I'm healing," I whisper quietly. "I'm healing."

Things are different in the months that follow—most of all me. I'm becoming more connected with my higher self. I'm becoming more loving toward myself. I don't fight with my body as much. I'm realizing how limiting the voices in my head often were. I'm learning to be more tender, gentler with myself. My pain is still insurmountable some days, but my soul is now close enough to answer back when my body speaks to me.

I need you, it says.

I'm here, I reply. *I love you. You're so beautiful, you're whole.*

I look into the mirror and let my eyes visit my scars like they're landmarks. I can see more beauty on my own naked skin than I ever have in any pink sunset and I speak it myself. I remember the affirmations:

"I am not broken, I am whole, I am loved, I am love."

When I feel vulnerable and the stories of pain and envy come back, I don't shame myself. I have shadows and I welcome them in, I try to treat them with grace and tenderness. They are a part of me—without them I wouldn't be whole.

When fear shows up, I say, "Hello, fear, thank you for coming here and trying to protect me. I'm going to buckle you in for the ride, but love is driving this bus."

When envy shows up, I remind myself, "Sweet Ruthie, I know that you sometimes worry that you are being forgotten. You think there's not enough love, money, and jobs in the world for all of us, but there is. It is abundant and it is everywhere. Remember, love is what's driving this bus."

In this season, I start to feel true love for myself, but I'm still learning how it is that I need to be loved. I still have more work to do. I begin to welcome my shadows instead of trying to push them away because of my shame, but I know that I need to explore them deeper.

Nicole Sachs is a fiery little woman from Delaware. I spot her as soon as she walks through the door of the restaurant. She's delicate-looking, like a china doll, but she has the energy of a lioness and I can feel her in front of me before she even makes it past the hostess stand. She spoke on a friend's podcast and I felt an immediate closeness when I heard her voice. Nicole is a therapist, a mother, and a writer. She suffered from a chronic, incurable physical ailment and she healed. I asked my friends if they could put us in touch and I called her right away.

We slide into a curvy vinyl booth next to a roaring fireplace that's totally gratuitous in Los Angeles. Even in February, it's seventy-five degrees outside.

"I really do believe that I can help you." Her empathetic, piercing eyes are glued to mine. Nicole believes that in many cases, chronic pain is the result of burying chronic emotional pain and she's developed a practice that helps people re-embody, repair the fractured mind-body connection that can occur when we bury our traumas.

"I'm ready," I tell her.

Nicole doesn't waste any time. She speaks quickly and drinks her lemon water quickly and teaches me quickly, but with love. I've never been a good student, but I try to be. She tells me that human beings have primitive wiring, that all of us fancy people wandering the world with our noses in our phones are still built like Neanderthals. We have one job here on earth: to survive. The problem is that survival can take a toll on *life*.

Nicole says that often in order for us to survive, our brains are wired to choose between what hurts and what hurts more in a moment of peril.

"Sometimes," she says, "during trauma, we disconnect from an experience emotionally to survive it physically."

"Disembodiment," I say. I feel the distance between my mind and my body—I've felt it for a long time. I think about smiling big at my daddy's funeral. I think about the accident.

She looks across the table at me and nods, glad that I'm keeping up, and adds, "But your body hangs on to all of it. And it hurts."

I watch her eyes get big and excited now. She tells me that my body has been asking me to pay attention, using physical pain as a kind of alarm bell. If I'm able to release my emotional pain, she thinks I might be able to release my physical pain as well.

I let it sink in and think about what my body has been saying to me:

I'm tired.

I need you.

I'm hurting.

But I didn't listen. I've been looking outside myself for direction instead of inward, putting all my hope in surgeries and medicines, in other people, but never in myself.

Nicole gets up from the booth. Before she leaves she talks to me about JournalSpeak, the practice she designed to help people let go of deep, repressed trauma. She teaches me the first step: making lists. I still love making lists.

I make lists so that I can remember. But the things I need to remember may be the ones I wish I could forget the most.

I wake up earlier than normal on Tuesday, back in Nashville. I get a glass of water and take a breath that seems to shake all the way in and all the way out. I decide to go through the exercise in my bedroom and sit down cross-legged on top of the covers. I let my eyes fall shut and try to connect with the Divine, the earth, and the sky.

"Show me where it hurts," I say with my eyes closed.

I take out my black Walgreens notebook and create three lists like she taught me. The first is titled "Childhood." I write down anything painful I can remember from when I was a little girl. It feels like nonsense.

Playground

Mom

Can't read/not smart

Bathtub

White dance at Jackson Hall

257

The next list is called "Present Day," and contains anything that comes up from ages eighteen until today. It doesn't matter if the things seem small—if I remember, Nicole says, they're important. I breathe in and continue:

Headaches
College. Binge eating.

I'm surprised when I think of it. For years, I convinced myself that college was a happy time, but the words arrive on the page and I remember. I was numbing my pain with food, overconsuming, then dieting. I was isolating and then showed up with a smile on my face.

I keep going, and one by one, painful memories I thought had disappeared return to me.

Jack and Allie
The church
US politics
Infertility
Daddy's death

And on and on. I feel myself wanting to drift away. My mouth is dry and my heart is beating too fast. I take another sip of water and continue. The third list is "Personality," all the masks I feel I must wear to feel safe in the world, to be loved and accepted:

Needs affirmation
Smiles when in pain

Tries to be good and accepted
Codependent

The lists can go on and on, but this is where I stop. The messy little scrawls look harmless on the paper, yet they hold so much weight for me, weight I've always felt but never really understood. I stare at the little crooked blue words knowing that they're the gateway to pain, to darkness, anger, shame, ugliness—things I've never, ever allowed myself to feel, let alone express.

Next, I grab my computer. I'm supposed to write about the things from the list for twenty minutes every day, say the things I've never given myself permission to say or release, things that weren't "good" that I've always felt but repressed. I'm nervous. I set the timer for twenty minutes, open my computer, and go.

Something comes over me. I place my fingers on the keys and they move. I don't even have to think. The words on the list that are screaming the loudest open massive, gaping wounds I forgot that I even had:

I'm nine years old next to my beautiful mom, feeling like I'm not pretty enough.

I'm watching Jack's eyes, a shade of brown I'll never forget, glow wildly for Allie.

I'm watching myself talking from a stage to a large group of people and wanting to feel their love, craving it like a drug.

I hear myself moan and cry; I hear the keys hammering and hammering and hammering away. The timer goes off. I don't look at what made it from my brain to the screen. Nicole told me not to. I just select it all and delete it. I continue the practice every morning.

Little by little, I feel released. Some days when I write I scream. Others, I'm so overcome with grief that I can barely breathe. I call people horrible, vile names and I weep, unearthing the profound ache of living in a world without my daddy, without a partner, without my own children. I give myself permission to feel freely and deeply, to look into my own shadows without fear or shame and also to bask in my light without feeling undeserving of warmth. After I go off on somebody or something and let go of the pain that connects me to them, I perform a love meditation, constructing a beautiful new bridge from my soul to theirs. I get still again, cover myself in love and grace, and then I send it on to whomever it was I was angry with. I imagine a chain of little heart bubbles. As the weeks go on, I begin to feel a peacefulness in my body.

After two months, I can look back at Jack with love. He stuck by me and supported me when I was in agony. I'm grateful to him and I'm grateful for us. We were just babies. We did our best, and we were dealing with so much. I can look back at the church with love too. I see the way it tried to protect me, love me, and shelter me from what it believed were evils and hold me close. The Christian church gave me order, and as my life circumstances pushed me through disorder, once I was able to confront the hurt I felt during those years, it led me to examine what it was I really did believe.

I recognize that I suffered a major spinal cord injury. I know my neck has more in common with a toaster oven than it does with a regular neck, but as I release emotional trauma, I begin to feel physical pain lift away. I can walk in my neighborhood. I can hold my friends' children. I can travel. I talk about healing because I'm finally beginning to believe in it. I still feel pain, but I also feel

peace and release and I'm in awe. The pursuit of a beau
once drove me to move and see and do, but it begins to call me
toward quiet and stillness.

For the first time in my life I start meditating daily. I was always afraid to be still; the pain screamed too loud in the quiet
and I never thought I could handle it, but as I trust in myself and
stay present, I realize the divinity in me speaks even louder. I start
seeing the divinity in all of us, in everything that Mother Nature
touches, from the dirt to the mountaintops. I try to go to her
church daily, grounding my feet in the earth and feeling a sense of
oneness and harmony with the world. I stop trying just to serve
others and instead try to learn from them. I try as gracefully as I
can to learn about racism, human rights, my own privilege, and
inclusivity. I want to use my voice and my platform to advocate
for voices that aren't being listened to. I have so much to learn.

I think about the oneness of us all, of everything. I want to explore it deeper. It's Holy Week and I'm at a monastery in rural
Kentucky surrounded by a thick evergreen wood. The birds are
loud here, cackling crows with shiny blue-black wings and yellow
finches that can't sing very well at all but try anyway, just like I do.
I don't say anything back to them as they whistle at me, because I
came here for complete silence. The idea of a silent retreat is scary
to me at first. I love to speak, I do it for a living, but now I know
the truth that can be found when you just stop and listen.

My room is small and simple: a single bed with a thin blue
blanket, a desk made of buttery blond wood, and an unadorned
cross stuck to the wall. In the mornings, I meditate, I do my

JournalSpeak as quietly as I can, and I stretch my body. I'm surprised by how open it feels, how gracefully I move when shame and fear aren't tugging at my muscles. At noon, I have my soup and bread and then I play in nature. Mother Earth has been one of my greatest teachers. I missed her when I was living in my bed; we have so much lost time to make up for.

I walk outside into a drizzle on my third day of silence. The woods are out back. I'm not sure how far they go, but there are a lifetime's worth of journeys to take in them, dozens of trails, each with its own ever-changing secrets: a network of skinny brooks, a tree as wide around as the house I grew up in, a family of anxious brown rabbits trying to disappear against the dirt. Today, I take a new path and though I don't know where I'm going, I feel safe, held close by the Divine, at home and connected to my body. Occasionally, another silent seeker passes by me on the trail. We nod and continue our respective soul searches, steps sinking into the mulch and grounding us to the earth.

There's a small shack where you can stop to pray under an oak tree. It's made of half very old lumber and half very old stone. I step inside and light a stick of incense, taking a moment to watch the smoke and smell curl into the air, pass through the open door and drift up in little ribbons toward the wet canopy. I think about healing.

For such a long time, I was searching for a cure: a good husband, a job, a pill, a surgery, a path to God, a path to enlightenment.

"Fix me. Make me better," I used to pray.

The words left my body more times than I can count, but what I needed more than anything was to hold on to them, to send them inside. It was never the cure that I needed; it was the healing, the spiritual and emotional peace, the connection between body and soul, the acceptance. Blue and golden flecks of sunlight sneak through the gaps in the walls as I stand and think. I remember living in my bed and I can hardly believe where I am and what I'm doing. I never imagined I'd have the physical, financial, and personal freedom to experience the world this way, to really pursue healing on my own terms.

Thank you. I look up and say it without releasing a word.

Drizzle gives way to sun. I leave the shack and continue up the path.

I go through the woods a little while longer, and then a burst of too-early summertime heat welcomes me into a broad clearing. Young golden flowers have opened all around and the clouds look like packing peanuts glued to the sky. In one direction the flowers stretch from the edge of the woods to the horizon, in the other they thin to grass, then to dust; the terrain beyond grows tall and rugged. My eyes find a path that snakes up between two soft peaks, more than hills but less than mountains, steeper still than any I've ever tried to climb before. I don't feel any fear, just peace, and I start on my way up, letting the body I once gave up on carry me higher and higher.

I listen to my body as I dodge plate-shaped rocks and twigs on the ground, but it has nothing to say. It's silent and joyful, like the rest of me. The muscles in my legs tighten and release, tighten and release, letting go of a little more fear, a little more grief with each step. I taste sweat on my lips and feel my lungs grow bigger with breath than I thought they could. I keep going up, up, up and feel the sunshine sloughing off years of old stories and traumas.

Finally, the ground levels. I've arrived.

What I would once have called barren feels instead like a place filled with promise. I walk almost to the edge of the ridge, left right, left right, and the smell of a hundred different flowers, of my own sweat and the minerals under my feet, hits my nose at once, a perfume that can't ever be bottled. I sit, body cradled in the most exquisite afternoon light. Held in that same light, the world stretches out in front of me, expansive, soaked in love, abundant with truth. I look out into the vista and behold everything in the glow: the monastery, the flowers, every animal and plant and human underneath the sky. It seems limitless. I imagine it illuminating my mom, my brothers, Jack, and Laura Treppendahl. I imagine the light falling across my daddy's smiling face. I think about him for a while. I always do in the beautiful places I go. Fat tears, part grief, part gratitude, slide down my skin and become a part of the earth beneath me. I weep as quietly as possible.

I wonder if he can see me, if he has a spot up front in the colossal, never-ending sky. I look down at my hand and remember the way it felt wrapped in his. I try to remember the last time we held on to each other but I can't.

I wish so badly that he could know me now. The last time we saw each other I was consumed with pain, living in my bed, and hopeless. Today, I climbed halfway to the clouds and I'm consumed with joy. I keep my eyes closed, stay still, trust in the universe, and hope for a sign of him. Somewhere.

22

Home

There's the journey of healing, the work of it, the treacherous climb toward peace. Then there's the magic of it.

We're at Tim's house staring up at the twinkling boughs of the Christmas tree. My niece Lucy is dancing and singing a pop song she probably shouldn't be listening to.

"She's just like you were," my mom says, smiling.

She's right. I watch Lucy for a moment, shaking her little hips as hard as she can, trying to boogie her way out of bedtime.

Laura and Libby laugh in the kitchen. The big kids practice cheerleading moves and baseball swings out in the yard. Lile and Tim half watch from the porch. It feels good to be home.

My mom and I are alone on the couch, talking. We talk often now, about life, my daddy, her hummingbird feeders, whatever floats into our minds. She's been one of my greatest champions, encouraging and embracing me in the most supportive and loving ways.

"Ru, have you ever done DNA testing?"

It's an odd question but her friends are all at the age where genealogy, like growing hydrangeas or entering pies in contests, becomes a hobby. I've done just about everything under the sun over the past year—tarot cards, sound baths, sweat lodges—so she's not wrong to assume that I spit into a test tube somewhere along the way.

"Several of your father's friends found out later in life that they had children, you know." She shrugs. "It was the sixties, boys were enlisting. It was a strange time."

Her eyes dart to the window as she speaks. I wonder if she expects to see my daddy walking across the yard toward her, the way he'd done so many times before. We both sit still in the silence for a while. The holidays are always a little gray without him.

"I actually have," I tell her, "but I've never logged in to my account or anything."

Ancestry.com sponsored a tour I spoke on earlier in the year and all the panelists got free testing. For a few minutes, I imagined that I was secretly an Italian noble, but then I forgot about it.

"You should. You never know." My mom's eyes, as gorgeous as ever, shine out into the tree line.

I don't log in. I go home and back to work and she doesn't bring it up again.

A few months later, I'm on the phone with an intuitive, a healer who taps into your energy from a distance and helps you better tap into it all yourself. I'm still trying to understand my place in the universe, my purpose. I still look everywhere for direction. She talks about my future, the book I'm writing, and where I'll be living in ten years. Then she tells me something I never expected to hear.

"I keep hearing 'missing brother.'"

My brain tells me it's crazy, but I think of my mom's eyes combing the garden for my daddy. Something in my soul tugs at me, insists that it's true. In the days that follow, it's as though I can feel him in the world, as though we were connected in spirit without ever meeting in the flesh.

It's May when I get the message.

A sweet woman writes me from Oxford, Mississippi, where I went to school.

"My husband matched with you on Ancestry.com. I believe that you're closely related to him."

I give her my phone number and wait. It rings less than an hour later.

"Do you know why I'm calling?" His name is David. His voice is a mix of Tim's gentleness and Lile's enthusiasm for absolutely everything.

"Yes," I tell him. "You're my brother."

Talking with him is wildly exciting and deeply comforting, like going away to somewhere you've been a hundred times and know that you love. His birth mother was eighteen years old when she visited LSU. It was 1965. My father was a college junior and she was a high school senior. They met at a fraternity house. She got pregnant and put the baby up for adoption. My daddy had no idea.

My father finished school and went to Vietnam. She went to college in Arkansas. David was adopted by a college professor at the University of Mississippi. He lived there most of his life and went to Ole Miss in Oxford, just like I did. I wonder if we've met before or shopped at the same grocery store, if we ever chose the same patch of grass at the Grove to lie down on. We've been to many of the same places, it turns out. We've been inches away from meeting for most of my life.

David sent his daughter, Mary Halley, to Camp DeSoto, the safe place I spent all my summers, where the air smells like sap and burnt marshmallow. As a college student, she was a counselor just like I was. She knew and loved all my nieces, who were her first cousins. She helped shy Kitty make friends and cut up her dinner into the right-size pieces. A few summers later, Mary Halley got a job at the boys' camp where my nephews go, and where Tim works summers as the doctor. They saw each other almost daily, waving across the cafeteria and nodding on the paths through the forest. Tim stayed up with her in the infirmary when she got a stomach flu, tying her matted hair back and sitting with her as she hugged the toilet, both totally unaware that they were uncle and niece.

Years later, she invited Tim's entire family to her wedding. They sat in the pews, smiling broadly at David as he walked his daughter down the aisle.

Time fades away from us as we talk. I scroll through the pictures on Facebook. He looks more like my daddy than any of us— the way he stands, the way he crosses his legs and seems to jump out from the photographs, his personality too big to be caught on camera. I tell him my story, about the accident, my pain, the medicine that made me lose myself. I recall the grief of losing my—our—daddy and he recalls the grief of losing his son.

The day David found me on Ancestry.com was the sixth anniversary of his son William's death; it was an accidental drug overdose. He died in Nashville like my daddy did, not ten miles from my house. I feel the Divine lay its hands on both of us, hundreds of miles apart as we speak, as a connection we'd both imagined materializes. We talk about pain, about what it is to lose yourself in it, to find yourself beyond it, about the hard lessons that come in learning to honor it. David tells me that he's started a wellness center at Ole Miss in honor of his son for drug and alcohol education and support, and suddenly I feel my precious Laura Treppendahl. I remember getting the call when she was killed by a drunk driver at Ole Miss. I think about her big bright eyes and how proud she'd be to know what my brother was doing. I feel her lay her hands on us too. None of it is accidental.

We get off the phone at dusk, when the sky is like artwork, pink and purple cloud dots with a squeeze of orange. I call my brothers and my mom: none of them are as shocked as I expect they'll be. Tim can't believe that they'd met before and Lile can't believe that they hadn't yet. My mom is peaceful, grateful to have another piece of my daddy in the world. We make plans to welcome David home.

A month later, we gather on our family farm in St. Francisville, my daddy's happiest place on earth, where he plowed his garden with his mule, buried his favorite dogs, and raised his children. Now it's where Tim and Laura raise theirs.

David had come to see me in Nashville a few weeks before. I was blown away by his face, his mannerisms, the way he held court with all my friends and captivated the room just like my father would. I felt unconditional love when we stood out on the curb of my house and held each other for the first time. It was like I had a piece of my daddy's love again, and now, right next to my daddy's garden, I watch that love grow wild.

I look out into the yard and watch my brothers, the three of them side by side, telling jokes and releasing enormous roars of laughter. I watch their children playing together and blow kisses to David's nine-month-old grandbaby, my daddy's first great-grandchild, perched peacefully on his mama's hip. I close my eyes for a moment.

Thank you, I say silently to the universe. *Thank you so much.*

We line up on the lawn for a family photo: me, my brothers, too many nieces and nephews to count, my mother, a bushel of cousins and friends, and I smile. We've come together to celebrate one another, the gift and collective strength of family, a family larger and farther reaching than any of us had ever known. My father and William are the only ones not here, but I know, I trust with all of me, that they were the forces that brought us together.

I sling my arm over the shoulders of David's daughter, my newfound niece, Mary Halley, as the camera on the tripod whirs and blinks and I peek down at her pregnant belly, life flourishing beautifully before my eyes. I'm floating over the farm in St. Francisville on a dream cloud. Pain is small and far away from us. It's still there—it always will be, but so will the magic and the miracles and the joy. Everything that happened did so for a reason. It happened to bring me home, to my family and to myself. It helped me see beyond the stories in my head; it helped me seek deeper truth and love earnestly. It led me to make peace with the God I thought had abandoned me and trust in the Divine, the love that had always been pouring down over me even when I couldn't see it. It pours down over all of us.

The line is noisy. The brand-new brothers can't stop laughing and telling stories, and the children are itching to get back to their games. My mom is smiling broadly with the deepest sense of pride. We stand under a sky that seems to stretch wider than the face of the earth we stand on. It's brilliant and beautiful, but on this day it can't compete with what's unfolding beneath it.

I see the red ants marching in another direction, away from me. I know they may come back. Healing isn't a process you complete—it's a journey you are on for a lifetime. I'm still journeying, just like anyone else.

The sun feels warm on my face and I hear my daddy's voice.

Home is all it says. It's all that needs to be said.

The camera's shutter flickers.

I'm awake but I keep my eyes closed, letting just enough light in to remind me that I'm home, that I always will be.

Author's Note

A year and a half ago when I sat down to write, I couldn't even sit at a desk. My brain barricaded me in physical pain to keep me from beginning this emotional journey. Brick by brick, the barriers began to come down, the stories began to unravel, the pain began to lift away.

Healing is not linear and neither is the journey I'm on. I have days where I feel so much love for myself, where I'm so in touch with the Divine and so connected to my world, and I have *other* days where I cuss at the person who cut me off in traffic, judge every person who walks by, and feel so impatient that I want to crawl out of my skin. I can go from meditating and sending love out into the universe to wanting to flip off a politician on TV. Healing is work and I don't always want to do the work. I don't always want to JournalSpeak, I don't always feel gratitude. I can sulk, shut down, and isolate with the best of them. More often than I'd like to admit, I want to climb back into my bed (she still calls me) and curl up with all the Real Housewives and all the peanut butter M&M's. But I ask for help and I stay very connected to my community, and the beautiful thing is, I have tools now to make those days easier and come back to my truth more quickly. The more of this extraordinary loving, healing work that I do, the better I get at it.

I don't know what your journey looks like but I do know that we're all on one. It can be crazy hard one minute and crazy beautiful the next. It never has to be perfect—I don't think any journey worth taking is. Mine sure isn't.

It has taught me a lot, though. Because pain is universal, I believe that healing is possible. I'm not talking about perfection, about waking up one day in remission, sober, or pain-free; I'm talking about finding peace and acceptance within yourself, a sense of home in your body and spirit. I have days where I forget everything that I've learned, where I crawl back into bed and sob. It isn't all peaks—there are valleys and there are deep, dark pits. I don't believe that our pain has to be wasted, though. I like thinking of all my painful, sorrowful moments as though they are not happening to me, but for me. Every breakdown is another opportunity for a breakthrough, another invitation to explore deeper, to journey further, to help someone along as they start on their own path. We need each other. In therapy they say that the opposite of addiction is connection. We were not meant to do this on our own. We need to heal in community, to be mirrors of truth and love to each other when the crazy person in our head is telling us so many limiting, effed-up stories.

Thank you for making space for this story. I'm honored and so incredibly grateful that you've chosen to travel so far with me. Now, close the book. Forget my name, forget my story—direct all the love, energy, and time you gave to me to yourself. You don't need me. This love, healing, and divinity is all inside you! You were never broken—you are good and whole and loved. You are love! Keep journeying until you believe it. You're so deserving!

I'm just gonna moonwalk out of here now so that you can get started.

Acknowledgments

The fact that this book exists feels utterly impossible, and it would not have been possible without the incredible love and support of my family and friends.

Thank you, Jennifer Walsh, for seeing me and believing in me.

Margaret Riley King, my beautiful agent/friend/sister, thank you for having faith in me way before I did. I love you so much.

Thank you to Lauren Spiegel, my wonderful editor, and to the whole Simon & Schuster family.

Shannon Miller, sweet sister, none of this would have been possible without you. Thank you for going on this crazy journey with me.

Thank you to my amazing friends, who have loved and supported me through all my ups and downs. My precious chosen family, Amber Sannan and Adi Brock, you are my lifelines and I don't know what I would do without you. You are my first calls when anything beautiful or painful happens. I thank God for you both constantly.

Thank you to Katie Moessner, my guide, my teacher, my best friend, my memory, you have always seen me and loved me so fully, and to Leslie Hill, you have never wavered in your love for me. I adore you. I'm so grateful Tupac brought all of us together at Camp DeSoto.

Katherine Carpenter and Debbie Taylor, I will never forget the way you showed up for me in my darkest hours. I am forever and ever grateful to you both.

Sean Brock, Micah Sannan, Claire Zinnicker, Raven Lewis, Jean-Vianney Philippe, and Christine Owenell, you have all played such beautiful roles in my becoming. Thank you so much for standing by me. I love you.

Jedidiah Jenkins, best friend, soul mate. I love you with all of me.

Thank you to my dear Sophia Bush for introducing me to Jennifer Walsh and opening up this amazing door. Thank you for believing in me and caring for me; it means more than you know.

Brian Daniel, thank you for loving me so well as a teenager, and I'm so glad it was you holding my hand the night that changed my life forever.

Thank you to my darling Frannie. I thought of you constantly while writing this book. This is for you, my precious sister. You are filled with grace, tenderness, and beauty, and I adore you.

Ann Patchett, my dear friend and mentor, thank you for seeing me instantly, supporting me always, and loving me so well. I am so deeply grateful for you.

Miles Adcox, my precious brother, you have loved and supported me in ways that leave me speechless. I can never repay you for all you have done for me. I am eternally grateful for you and your friendship.

Thank you to my ex-husband for sticking by me through some of the toughest years of my life. I am deeply appreciative of you and your beautiful family.

Everyone at Onsite and Milestones, you changed my life and helped bring me back home to myself. Thank you for the incredible work that you do.

Daddy, thank you for gifting us with your son David Magee. I am so grateful for my brother and to have another piece of you in my life. David, I didn't know how deeply I was missing you and your precious family until we met that very first time. I'm so excited for all our future memories.

Mom, your heart contains the most breathtaking, life-changing, unadulterated beauty I've ever known. Thank you for teaching me what it is to mother. I know you had to learn a lot of that love on your own, and you embody it like no other.

Lile, my bubby, my first true love, my protector, the face that pops into my head whenever I hear the words "unconditional love," thank you for delighting in me. You've made me feel valued and treasured from the moment I was born.

Tim, "T-Bird," you're the clearest picture of divine love I've ever seen in this world. Knowing you is knowing God and grace, humility and healing, pure, unspoiled goodness. Thank you for teaching me.

Laura, you've never *not* been my sister. Your love has nurtured me my whole life and I'm in awe watching it nurture the six sweet souls you've brought into this world. You love them exactly as they are and you love me exactly as I am. You're the greatest gift.

Libby, I couldn't have dreamed of a better partner for Lile. You were the missing piece of our puzzle. You gave me the feeling of home when I thought I'd lost it forever. You made me laugh when I could hardly speak and you showed me radical love when I thought I was unlovable. You're the best boy mom ever and I adore you.

ACKNOWLEDGMENTS

Mary Margaret, Lile, Betsy, Rhodes, Kitty, Tim, Parks, Michael Patrick Quinn, and Lucy, you've inherited a legacy of love, you have your papa's eyes, your parents' hearts, and a whole wide world waiting for you. You were each created so perfectly and so uniquely and there is no greater joy for me than seeing your stories unfold. I love you, remember your manners, always look out for the little guy.

About the Author

Ruthie Lindsey is a speaker, cohost of the *Unspoken* podcast, and prominent social media figure who challenges audiences to seek joy and find the healing that is inside all of us. She lives in Nashville, Tennessee. This is her first book.